Revamp

Your Health

Lose body fat and gain confidence, health, happiness, and strength through 6 easy steps to total body health and wellness

By Stephanie Walker

With submissions from Erik Walker and others

Blue River Health and Wellness
Harrisonburg, VA

Purple Cider Publishing
Walker-Wimer Group LLC
1743 Kingston Court
Harrisonburg, VA 22801

Ordering Information:
Quantity sales. Special discounts are available on quantity purchases by corporations, associations, and others. For details, contact the publisher at the address above.
Orders by U.S. trade bookstores and wholesalers. Please contact Erik Walker erik@erikwalker.net

Printed in the United States of America

ISBN-10:1-943975-02-7
ISBN-13:978-1-943975-02-0

First Edition

Nutrition and Hydration

Exercise and Movement

Sleep Hygiene

Energy and Time Management

Stress Reduction

Personal Growth and Development

Inside *REVAMP*, you'll find the keys that will help you learn how to eat better in a way that works best for YOU. You'll build routines that help manage your stress and balance your energy, learn strategies for time management, and you'll develop exercise routines you'll stick with. Best of all, you'll start to build the confidence in yourself that will lead you down a path of lifelong success for both you and your family. *Finally,* you can start meeting the goals you've been setting for yourself.

"Stephanie understands both the logic and science behind eating and training for athletic performance. While she's been coaching me, I've had a PR in every lift and gained new abilities in gymnastic skills. If you're willing to put in the work, Stephanie can show you the way."
Lyndsey Martin

"July 2015 I was desperate. I started researching strength training and weight loss and came across Stephanie's article "Are You Under-eating? Overeating? How Many Calories Do You Really Need?" I read the article and then I read her bio and thought "this is me and she gets it!" I reached out to Stephanie and told her all my issues and frustrations. 12 weeks later I had gained a few pounds [of muscle] but I was down 2 dress sizes! At 44 I am in the best shape of my life!"
Jill Evans

Stephanie is a health coach and fitness instructor who knows what it's like to start from scratch to change her life. After losing over forty pounds post-college by following the six pillars of health upon which she wrote in REVAMP, she now coaches others who are looking to make the same changes. She has blogged about her journey on strongfigure.com, and has built blueriverhealth.com in order to reach out to those who desire one-on-one health coaching. Stephanie has been featured in the Washingtonian, Fitfluential, Fitbloggin', and is a feature writer for wodnationgear.com's *Whiteboard*. Stephanie is also the co-author of ***The Total Health and Fitness Makeover***, and founder and co-owner of Strongfigure.com and BlueRiverHealth.com.

Preface:

No matter who you are or what goal you're working to achieve, true health is not just nutrition and exercise. To be happy, confident, and successful; your health is a combination of your mental, physical, and emotional state. I believe in coaching the WHOLE you. And this book, REVAMP, serves as the model of both my personal and my company mission: coach the whole person--not just part.

REVAMP is more than just a nutrition or a health book. REVAMP contains a built-in workbook with easy to understand actionable steps that help walk you through the entire process of starting your very own total body and mind transformation. REVAMP is built on statistics, research, methods, and perhaps most important--experience.

I've worked incredibly hard to transform my own health over the past 15 years. I come from a place of using food for comfort and not knowing how to exercise; to overcoming insecurities, dieting problems, and finding a way to live a normal, happy, healthy, lifestyle--permanently. To give you a bit of my back story—

- I gained 40+ pounds in college.
- I didn't know how to lose weight so I yo-yo dieted and screwed up my metabolism.
- I started exercising, mostly with cardio, and ended up over-exercising, under eating, and worsening my already poor metabolism.
- I knew nothing about nutrition or carbs, good fats and bad, low fat vs full fat, or how much protein to eat.
- I learned everything the hard way.

Over the past 15 or so years, I can without a doubt say that I've tried everything. I've learned more about my body than I ever thought possible. I learned the right way to eat, the better way to train, and how to regain the confidence I lost early in my 20s while struggling with my weight issues. Within this time in my life, I even found my husband.

Transforming my health has led me to find a whole new purpose in life and it's helping others. I desperately want others to know that if I can come from a background of knowing absolutely NOTHING, and transition into a career of coaching others, then it's possible for anyone to change. That's why REVAMP exists. It's to show that with a little patience and a lot of dedication, YOU can make the change you've always to make in your life. And most of all, I want this book to teach you that nutrition and exercise alone aren't the only ways to find what you've lost or to reclaim your health. Elements like sleep, stress reduction, proper hydration, time management, and learning how to build your confidence are the missing elements that most health coaches forget to mention.

To those of you who have struggled and are tired of trying all the fads that claim to work but leave you feeling failed and depressed, I am excited to help you find the missing elements that YOU need to find the success you've been searching for.

Please find our very special group on Facebook and join us in the conversation of reclaiming health and wellness in our lives. Connect with me, with my husband Erik, with others just like yourself, and we'll help you get through the bad days, celebrate the good, and answer the questions you've been trying to ask for far too long.

Welcome to REVAMP, and we look forward to the transformation you're about to embark upon.

Table of Contents

Introduction:

I believe there are six important pillars of total body health and wellness and that no one is truly healthy until he or she has devoted time to working on each.

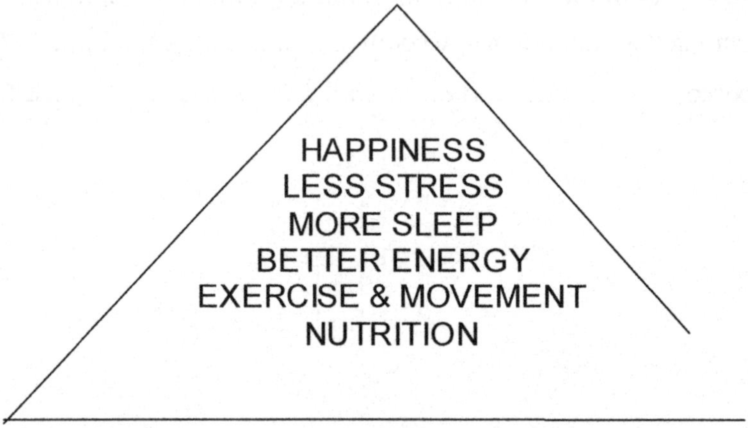

The Blue River Total Body Wellness Open Delta: because you are ALWAYS working on YOU.

1. **Nutrition and Hydration** -- *Health begins on the inside!* Nutrition is on the bottom of our pyramid because we believe it is the base. Understanding food and YOU is essential to having energy, moving well, sleeping better, feeling emotionally stable, and providing the vitamins and minerals your body needs for fighting disease and taking care of itself. Nutrition is the foundation for better health.

2. **Exercise and Movement** -- *Learn how to become and stay active, for life!* Nutrition may be

the foundation of your house, but every house needs walls. Being active and mobile is essential for a happy, confident, energetic, and longer life!

3. **Sleep Hygiene** -- *Our bodies can't function optimally without sleep!* Poor sleep hinders every circumstance of life. From the choices we make over foods, all the way to developing life-threatening diseases, sleep is one of the most critical elements of health.

4. **Energy and Time Management** -- *Make your life work for you--not the other way around.* We live in a busy, busy world. Being tired and not having the time or energy to spend with those you love will not lead you to a path of happiness or renewed health. Being able to manage your life, your family, and still have energy in the process is a lot simpler than you think...and healthier too.

5. **Stress Reduction** -- *Letting go of unwanted stress improves health instantly.* Simply, stress kills. Who wants to be under tension his or her whole life? No one! No one likes to be constantly stressed and no one likes being around a person who is always stressed. Stress leads to poor health, disease, and yes--a shorter life span.

6. **Personal Growth and Development:** *Building your confidence account is key for ultimate success!* At the tip of our pyramid, you'll find happiness. When you know what works best for your body and you understand how to manage your life, organize your priorities, reduce your stress, and eat great foods--you will be on the road to increased confidence and rejuvenated happiness.

Isn't that what we all want in the long run anyway? ***Happiness?***

REVAMP has been written to help you work on all six pillars of your health: the WHOLE you matters.

If at any point while you're reading this book you have any questions, please don't hesitate to contact us. You can best reach me on Facebook, or at blueriverhealth@gmail.com.

Even if you don't have any questions, we'd love for you to come by and say hello!

Your health should be your primary focus in life. When your health is optimal, your life functions optimally and that includes your relationships too! Look at the questions below and take a long hard look at your life as it stands right now.

- Do you get at least eight hours of quality sleep every night?
- Do you find yourself losing energy throughout the day?
- Do you eat the right foods at the right times?
- Do you know what foods work best for you? Which ones don't?
- Do you drink enough water each day or know how much to drink?
- Do you live an active lifestyle or a sedentary one?
- Do you have too much stress in your life?
- How are the relationships in your life?
- Do you find yourself constantly looking at life and/or people with a negative attitude?
- Are you happy and living your life with confidence or are you depressed and living with low self-esteem?

How do these answers make you feel? Go ahead; think about it for a moment. How do you feel right now about your life versus how you want to feel? How you wish you felt?

It's ok to feel a little down right now. Everyone has "that moment" where he/she realizes something needs to change. You're having that moment (or you've had it already) and that's why you're reading this book. This is a good sign! You're ready for change and many times, accepting this fact is the toughest part of starting a new journey.
Understanding and accepting the need for change is actually a transitional step your brain has made for you. You can't just make someone eat better or go to the gym because you want to, or you think he or she should. Each person must come to terms with his or her life, on her own, and accept the need for change, and most importantly, ***want*** to change. Because you're here right now, you've accepted the fact that you're ready. CONGRATULATIONS! The first step is complete.

Now, let's look at these questions from a different perspective:

- Do you want to look good and feel good--inside and out?
- Do you want to be stronger, fitter, and have more confidence?
- Do you want more energy in your day? Less stress?
- Do you just find yourself wanting to be happy?

If you said yes to at least one of these bullets, guess what? You're already taking steps towards better health and you should be proud of yourself! Because you're committing yourself to a lifetime of better health, you've already boosted your confidence and that's huge as far as continued success. So now that you've taken this step, what do you do next? How do you continue your path towards a lifetime of success and happiness? Looking good and feeling great?

You follow through. You learn how to become fitter, healthier, happier, and more confident about your life.

It's time--right now!--to REVAMP your life.

There is no better time than right now to make a change.

"Don't wait until everything is just right [...] There will always be challenges, obstacles and less than perfect conditions. So what. Get started now. With each step you take, you will grow stronger and stronger..." --Mark Victor Hansen

America is facing some serious health problems and they are almost all 100% preventable.

Obesity, heart disease, depression, having a lack of energy, being over-stressed and over-worked, underpaid, and underappreciated, eating fast food instead of healthy food...this has become the American lifestyle and it's leading us to serious disease and early death.

I don't know about you, but this is terrifying to me. People are tired. You may be one of them. You work all day, manage your family, try to manage your stress, put meals on the table, get a restless night's sleep, suffer from anxiety, have no confidence in yourself, and get very little exercise. You don't have time and possibly not enough funds for the extra gym membership and the organic salads--much less the energy for any of it--on top of everything else life throws at you.

Life shouldn't be this tough. Life doesn't have to be this tough.

So what gives?

The United States is a sedentary society with access to plentiful, rich, delicious foods. With our constantly advancing technological environment, many of us aren't as physically active as our ancestors once were, and the food that we can buy in supermarkets, restaurants, gas stations—let's just say we're not hard up for calories. Life is busier, we get exhausted, and food becomes more accessible--in a not-so-healthy kind of way.

In fact, it's a natural human instinct to eat a lot of delicious, calorie-dense foods and even avoid hard physical exertion. Our culture has since evolved, but our biology and physiology has not. And what happens when we let our advancement get in the way of our natural biology?

Simply, we need to exercise and prioritize our health. Our total health--body and mind.

According to a new study in the journal *Medicine & Science in Sports & Exercise,* researchers studied several sets of twins throughout their lifetimes. While half of the twins remained active throughout life, the ones who did not, had about seven more pounds of body fat, worse cardiovascular endurance, and insulin sensitivities that showed signs of early metabolic disease. "Not only were their bodies different; their brains diverged as well. The athletic twins had more gray matter (the information processing part of the brain), particularly in areas that controlled balance and motor function." Clearly, a lack of exercise may lead to poor health, disease, metabolic damage, and obesity.

Obesity

According to the CDC.org, obesity was more than common in 2014--it was serious and costly. More than one-third (roughly 78.6 million!) of U.S. adults were obese: at risk for serious life-threatening diseases.

Obesity-related conditions include heart disease, stroke, type 2 diabetes and certain types of cancer--some of the leading causes of preventable death.

It's not just that being obese is costing Americans like you and me a lot of money, but it's costing us our lives! Children are larger than they've ever been and are expected to live at minimal, five years less than that of their parents. And the baby boom generation? The life expectancy is declining.

We all need healthy insides to be able to live a longer, more fulfilling life. We need muscle mass, bone density, healthy organs, strong connective tissues, balance, strength, and coordination in order to age gracefully and with dignity, and NOT have to rely on our children to take care of us or worse, put us into nursing homes. We need confidence in our abilities, positive life behaviors that our children will emulate, less stress, more energy, and most importantly--happiness.

If you're not saving your own life yet, NOW is the time!

Why do you think so many people who sign up for gym memberships or go on diets, fail to get their desired results? Total body health requires more than just eating a few salads, upping your protein intake, and hitting the gym a few times a week. Even though nutrition and fitness make up a huge part of your health and physical fitness, usually programs fail because the parts lacking are the mental and emotional aspects. People actually sabotage their own work with a poor mental attitude.

How?

Because success isn't so much about "what to do" to reach goals; a lot of your success is going to come from the reasons you currently are UNsuccessful. To revamp your health, you're going to have to stop doing and thinking in ways harmful for your health. "Mindset" and "Motivation" are not always the same.

Total body health means accepting that you want a better life, knowing you need to change your habits, and understanding you're going to have good days, bad days, worse days, and days that make you want to give up. It's all about the *mindset*. Those who find success are the ones who don't give up. Those who turn their lives around are the ones who persist, wake up and try again, and those who don't beat themselves up on the inside when they have a bad day or even a bad week, month, or year.

Total body health means

- Accepting what you currently believe may not be true. The brain is incredible and your perspective in life is drawn off past experiences lodged in your brain. And guess what? Your body is connected to your mind. Your body does what the mind says. You need to accept that the past doesn't control your body and open your mind to new experiences.
- Gaining awareness of what your unconscious mind is saying so that you can increase the possibility of creating lasting change. What do your actions and behaviors--the ones you act out without really thinking--say about you? If you think you can't do something--you won't. You need to become aware of your thoughts--especially as they relate to your actions. Your body is going to follow your mind–wherever it goes.
- Becoming empowered by the reality that YOU control. When you control your perceptions you can change your perceptions and move yourself closer to the direction you want to be in.
- Adapting your mindset. Your mind is either set--fixed already on what you choose to believe--or it's changeable. And your mind is going to be either conscious or unconscious. You need to choose to be conscious of your thoughts and actions 100% of the time.

Total body health is a journey. And if you don't start appreciating the journey you have chosen, you're not going to reach your destination.

Six elements stand between you and your destination. You may already be practicing a few and are looking for help with the others. You may be a total health and wellness beginner and feel intimidated about tackling six new things in your already busy life. Don't worry! That's what this book is all about: teaching you how to incorporate each element in all aspects of your life--one at a time.

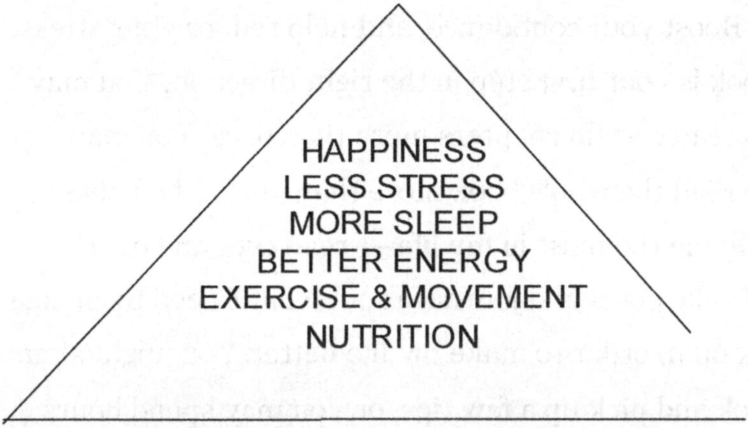

The Blue River Total Body Wellness Open Delta: because you are ALWAYS working on YOU.

1. Nutrition and Hydration -- *Health begins on the inside!*

2. Exercise and Movement -- *Learn how to become and stay active, for life!*

3. Sleep Hygiene -- *Our bodies can't function optimally without sleep!*

4. Energy and Time Management -- *Make your life work for you--not the other way around.*
5. Stress Reduction -- *Letting go of unwanted stress improves health instantly.*
6. Personal Growth and Development: *Building your confidence account and understanding YOU is key for ultimate success!*

Whether this list looks easy or intimidating, we want to walk you through each step. We want to increase your health. Boost your confidence, and help reduce your stress. This book is your first step in the right direction. You may have to read certain chapters more than once. You may have to read the whole book more than once. The books that help me the most in my life--I read over and over again. I take notes and journal about what I need to change or work on in order to make my life better. You might skim this book and pick up a few tips, or you may spend hours soaking up new knowledge. Whatever your goals are right now at this point in your life--that's what you'll do with this book: use it to help fuel your passion for whatever change you need right now.

The List

What's interesting about this list is that you probably already know that these are the elements you need more of in your life. I mean, that's why you're here. But how do you completely turn around a life that's consumed by stress, rushing from point A to B to C, picking up a fast food dinner, dropping off so-and-so at practice number one, squeezing in a 30-minute spin class, remembering to guzzle down enough water (with your vitamins of course), not forgetting to pick up both the kid at practice and your dry cleaning too (and/or your other kids), get everyone in bed for a halfway decent night's sleep, and wake up late to rush through the cycle again?!?!

Is this life *for real*?

How many people do you know who drink more than enough water each and every day, who also get 8+ hours of sleep, wake up early to organize the day, exercise, stretch, eat properly, read, meditate, etc.? You probably know several people who accomplish a couple of these important "musts" but I bet you don't know many who fit all six requirements into their schedule every day.

We all know that life just happens. Prioritizing things like grass-fed butter and yoga class sometimes take a back seat to convenience and excuses. But we're here to tell you not only how to re-shape your life, but why it's essential to rethink your priorities.

> *Start by doing what's necessary, then do what's possible, and suddenly you're doing the impossible. – St. Francis of Assisi*

Although there are only six steps to ultimate health and wellness, it's important to know that you'll have to work on each one-by-one, and it'll be close to impossible to achieve *any of them* without proper motivation. Therefore, before you read further, it's time to figure out your WHY. "What motivates or has motivated you to accept this change?"

Step One: What's your WHY?

Recently, I read this question posted in a Facebook group:

"I'm looking for some advice [...] that can help guide me or help me. I cannot follow through with anything....diet, exercise, [...]. Nothing sticks for more than a week or two. I want to exercise, I want to eat right and lose weight, I want all of these things but don't seem to have the motivation, willpower, or self-control to make it happen. Why???"

I wanted to shout through my iPhone: You just answered your own question with your last word: WHY!!!!!!

Sorry for the overuse of exclamation points, but I really want this to hit home with you. If you don't have your "why," you'll always find an excuse. You'll lose motivation when a bad day at work leaves you with a bottle of wine and cupcake in your hand. You'll lose your fight if you don't have a why. So that's what we've GOT to do before we can do anything else. You need to find your WHY.

Figure out what (or who) motivates you. Are you motivated by your significant other? Are you motivated by the thought of what your life could be if you improved your health? Are you motivated with the thought of being a role model for your children?

Finding your "WHY" might just be the hardest part of this whole journey. But once you're motivated, the rest becomes easy. Your "why" changes your mindset, fuels your motivation, and your motivation gets through each and every day.

So let's find that motivation.

Answer the following questions (and feel free to post your answers in our *Insiders* Facebook Group!) :

1. Why are you reading REVAMP?

2. Who motivates you to be healthier and fitter? And why?

3. For whom do you want to become fitter and healthier? Explain.

4. (The most important question) Visualize yourself: your life, those in your life, and your own happiness, ***after*** finding success with the six steps of wellness. What do you see?

5. What/Who is your WHY? And what or who is going to drive you through the days that make you want to give up?

Stuck on ideas? Here's my WHY:

When I first decided I needed to turn my life around, I saw this picture:

I was unhappy in life and in relationships. Emotionally I had been beaten down--by myself and by others. None of my relationships were healthy and even the ones that seemed fine, weren't right for me. Why? Because this wasn't ME.

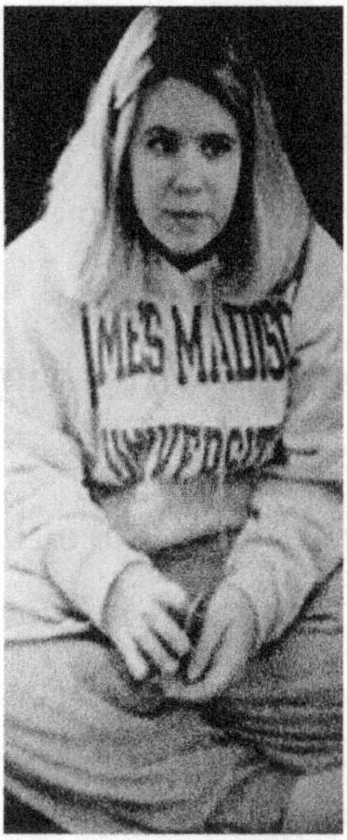

I saw this photo after my mom had taken it and I immediately knew that A) This was not the person I knew I could be and B) I also knew I wouldn't find the kind of happiness and respect I wanted out of life if I didn't change.

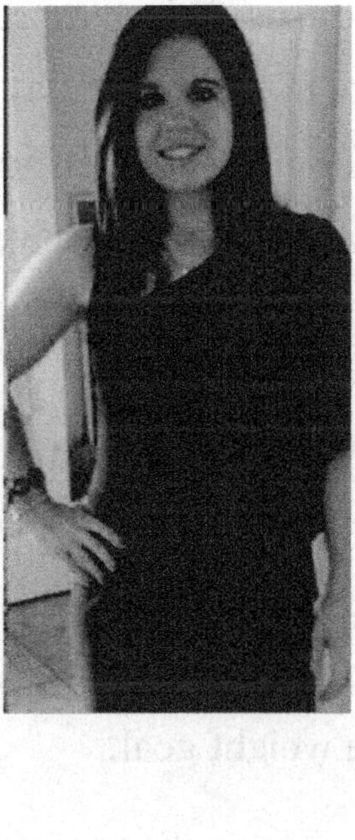

That became my why. I desired respect and I wanted to find the real me.

Knowing who I could become and

gaining the respect I knew I deserved out of life was all the motivation I needed to start my journey.

And I did. I found success, happy relationships, even better business ventures. I've published books and have found AND pursued my truest passions in life: helping and teaching others.

My "Why" is actually different now--and that's something that you can expect to happen to you as well. As your life starts to change, your "whys" can change too! Right now, my "why" is my family and my future—specifically my baby girl! I want to be her role model and teach her everything about growing up happy, strong, and confident. My health is better than ever, my confidence (the hardest part of my journey!) has improved tremendously, and my goal now is to live the life I have always dreamed of for my little girl: a life full of travel, adventure, love, happiness, and raising a wonderfully happy, healthy family. And I *really* want to make that possible for you too.

My "why" is continually evolving and you need to know that it's important to always have a "why." You don't just lose 50 pounds and go back to eating cupcakes and fast food--you must have a reason and a desire to *stay well*--not just meet a weight goal.

When I met my physical goals several years ago, my "why" became helping others--this simply makes me feel accomplished and important--almost like an "inner why." Wanting to be a role model for my daughter allows me to work on my personal growth and that's one of my biggest goals--being a better person and a healthy (mentally, emotionally, and physically healthy) source of inspiration for *any* person who needs me--especially my daughter. That means continual self-improvement. We are all works in progress with good and bad days. We've all made mistakes--whether it's a food mistake or life mistake. But if we have positive "whys" in our lives, we have reasons, desires, and the will to succeed.

If you haven't found it yet, take some more time to find your WHY before moving on. This may require some soul searching and even elimination of some of the negatives (relationships, habits, etc.,) in your life. But think about it carefully and really work to envision your future. Where will you be and what does your life look like when you meet your goals?

(PS: If you own the the StrongFigure *Total Health and Fitness Makeover Book* and/or *Workbook*, you can reference it for more motivational stories!)

Again, what's YOUR why?

NEXT: It's time to have a deeper conversation with yourself.

1. What past experiences may be holding you back or might try to challenge your mindset as you take this journey?

2. What do your current actions and behaviors say about you? Which ones are you going to change and how?

3. What perceptions of yourself would you like to change?

4. How will you plan to become conscious of your mindset so that your past thoughts, beliefs, and mistakes do not control your future?

Once you have found your WHY, and you've had a long conversation with the inner-you, you're ready to start your journey.

Hopefully by now you have identified your WHY. Now it is time to tackle your nutritional health.

Understanding food is easier than you probably think. It's also the most complex area in all of health and wellness. Oxymoron, huh?

Here's the simple part: We all need food in the form of carbs, fats, and proteins (macronutrients) to survive.

The complex part: Some people need more of these three macronutrients than others. Figuring out what works for YOU is going to be a challenging, yet FUN part of this new journey.

This chapter will teach you the basics plus all the important information you need about nutrition and hydration.

Revamping your nutrition isn't something that happens overnight. A lot of thought has to go into your goals, understanding your body, knowing what truly makes you happy, and building up your confidence enough to trust the process and push through the bad days. You may be able to skip around in this section, or you might find yourself reading it several times to really let the info sink in. No matter what, know that time and patience are key. Educate, experiment, don't be afraid to fail, and know that eating healthy is a lifestyle decision that you can't take lightly or look for quick fixes.

That said, let's start with the simplest topic: WATER.

Drink More Water!

The human body is composed of about 60-80% water. Fluids in the body--digestive, absorption, circulative, saliva, nutrient transports, and body temperature maintenance--is regulated by water. Water is crucial for various chemical reactions in the body.

Water is the most important and abundant compound in the human body and even accounts for approximately 73% of lean body mass. Staying hydrated is an absolute necessity for optimal health, mental function, and performance.

When looking at water through a weight loss eye, water allows your digestive system to function optimally, flushing the kidneys and keeping the total body hydrated--ultimately helping your metabolism to function better. And water even helps make your skin and overall appearance better.

Dehydration Causes:

- A lack of energy
- Improper removal of waste products from the body
- Pain in the body
- Gallstone formation
- Stress, depression, fear, anxiety
- Chronic Fatigue Syndrome

And Chronic Dehydration Can Lead To:

- Heart Disease
- Obesity
- Rheumatoid Arthritis
- Stomach Ulcers
- Hypertension
- Cancer
- Multiple Sclerosis
- Alzheimer's
- Fibromyalgia
- Migraines

Unfortunately, most people are NOT getting enough water daily. And those who are trying to "diet," sometimes end up hungrier from the dehydration symptoms felt from the lack of water and end up eating even more. Human beings need a sufficient amount of water to take care of the body and its functions--including appetite! The American College of Sports Medicine has reported that *"humans do not voluntarily consume sufficient water to maintain optimal fluid balance."* Sometimes, just a little bit more water can make the biggest difference in one's overall health.

If you're reading this because you want to improve your quality of life and become healthier, then water is going to be your first step. Water helps you become healthier, stronger, leaner, smaller, and happier.

Water can:

- Help control calories and promote weight loss by making you feel full. Since water-rich foods require more chewing, and are absorbed by the body at a slower pace, this allows you to feel full even while consuming less calories. And water metabolizes stored fat and suppresses the appetite! Here are some water-rich food sources worth adding to your grocery list:
    - Cucumbers
    - Leafy Greens, especially lettuce
    - Strawberries
    - Watermelon
    - Citrus Fruits
    - Celery
    - Full fat, plain yogurt
    - Papaya
    - Squash
- Water helps keep your muscles energized and ready for performance, and it also helps prevent cramps and sprains. Water helps keep the muscles and joints lubricated so you're less likely to get injured or feel pain. Not to mention it boosts

overall energy levels. In fact, a lack of water is the biggest indicator of daytime fatigue. A simple 2% drop in body water can cause memory problems, trouble with basic math, and difficulty focusing on a printed page or computer screen.

- Water keeps your skin looking fabulous as it helps prevent excess fluid loss. Dehydration can cause you to look older, wrinkled, and dry.
- Water helps your kidneys function properly—cleansing your body of toxins, preventing urinary tract infections—and helps your body maintain normal bowel function. Those who drink too little water are also at a higher risk for kidney stones.
- Water boosts your immune system and keeps you happy! Water enhances your mood and helps fight against the flu and other diseases. It even relieves and prevents headaches, migraines, and backaches--sometimes due to dehydration as well.
- Last, water increases your energy and relieves fatigue. Drinking water helps your brain think, concentrate, and focus better.

Did you know? A decrease in water will cause fat deposits to increase, while an increase in water can reduce them?

Did you know? Our thirst mechanism is so weak that most mistake it for hunger. One glass of water shut down hunger pangs for almost 100% of dieters studied.

How much water should you drink?

The "general" rule is this: The majority of us need to drink at the minimum, half our body weight in ounces of water every day to provide our bodies with the MINIMUM water requirements. A 150-pound person should drink a minimum of 75 ounces of water each day.

If you know how many calories you consume each day (or you have a pretty good estimate), a great hydration tip to follow is to drink 5 ounces of water per every 100 calories consumed. This ensures you're properly hydrated AND you have enough water to help your digestive system.

For serious athletes, 1-2 gallons of water per day is recommended.

And speaking of athletes, if you're exercising (or when you start exercising), experts agree that water actually works as a better energy and hydration source than carbs and sugar-filled sports drinks for most forms of moderate exercise.

Skip the beverages loaded with sugar!

Even though fruit juice contains natural sugar from fruits, when these drinks are processed, the sugars in the cell walls are released as free sugars, which are a leading cause in tooth decay, and these free sugars are non-nutritious or wasteful calories. Additionally, many fruit juices add sugar, glucose-fructose syrup, or high fructose corn syrup to their products to make them taste even sweeter.

Science Editor recently produced a study that revealed in a quarter of the fruit juice products tested, they found as much sugar as Coca-Cola.

Sugary Drinks May Lead to:

- A 31% greater risk for becoming obese
- A 30% higher risk of having a larger waistline
- A 25% higher risk of developing high triglycerides or high blood sugar
- A 32% greater risk of having low levels of good cholesterol
- A trend toward an increased risk of high blood pressure

Many health issues can be prevented or even sometimes cured just by replacing sugary drinks like juice and soda with a little more water.

Bonus! Top 7 Reasons to Drink Water Instead of Sodas:

1. Sodas dehydrate the body and the high sugar content steals more water from the body than the soda supplies. The high levels of phosphates steal vital minerals from your body, and a severe lack of minerals can lead to heart disease, osteoporosis, and many other diseases.

2. Soft drinks can remove rust. Think about that and your insides for a while.

3. Aspartame is found in diet sodas which are linked to a host of illnesses including depression, neurological disease, and insomnia--just to name a few. Also, drinking soft drinks--diet or not--lowers your immune system and keeps you from fighting illnesses!

4. Soft Drinks are VERY acidic, and they can eat through the liner of an aluminum can! They can also leach aluminum from the can if it sits on the shelf too long. Alzheimer patients who have been autopsied ALL have high levels of aluminum in their brains. Heavy metals in the body can lead to many neurological and other diseases.

5. Sodas interfere with digestion. Caffeine combined with high amounts of sugar can shut down the body's digestive process so that the body is essentially taking in NO nutrients from the food previously eaten, even food that is eaten hours earlier.

6. The insane amount of sugar in sodas causes your pancreas to produce an overabundance of insulin, which leads to a "sugar crash." And chronic elevation and depletion of sugar and insulin can lead to diabetes as well as other imbalance-related diseases. This is especially disruptive to growing children whereas an abundance of soda drinking tends to take place in our current society.

7. Soft Drinks do NOT quench your thirst, and they certainly do not quench your body's need for water. Denying your body the proper amount of water can lead to chronic cellular dehydration--a condition that weakens your body's immune system and the presence of minerals can lead to lifelong health problems.

Types of Water to Drink

- Tap Water is often referred to as drinking water since it is intended for drinking. Tap water may contain safe for human consumption additives such as fluoride, which is necessary for the health and growth of your teeth and gums.

- Distilled Water is highly purified water that filters out all contaminants and natural minerals. Because distilled water lacks these minerals it is generally not considered the healthiest water for human consumption.

- Purified Water has been purified to remove contaminants. Depending on the purification process used (carbon filtration, deionization, distillation, or reverse osmosis) the water, like distilled water, may also lack beneficial minerals.

- Spring Water comes from a natural source and it is often treated to reduce chemicals and other contaminants. Spring water by definition should contain healthy minerals but many bottled waters labeled as spring water do not necessarily come from a spring.

Recommendation: If you live in a municipal area that has safe drinking water, then drink it. If you feel the need to filter your water of dangerous contaminants then do so but just make sure you are drinking enough water!

The Question Everyone Asks: *"But I thought you could die if you drink that much water?!"*

There is a very rare condition called hyponatremia, which is caused by extreme water consumption that can actually be fatal. These cases often make the news and scare people away from drinking an adequate amount of water. However, these people are often drinking a CRAZY amount of water and doing activities that cause a tremendous amount of sweat–like running a marathon. Both of which would lead to loss of sodium, which leads to swelling of the cells and this can cause swelling in the brain–and that is bad. If you are running a marathon and plan on drinking four gallons of water, then you need to do some research on how to run a marathon. No expert will tell you to drink four gallons of water for such an activity. Extreme conditioning activities will require sodium supplementation through a product such as Drip Drop.

START RIGHT NOW!

Figure out how much water you need to drink daily and

start now. Don't put off your goals or say "I'll start tomorrow or next week." Take control of your situation by beginning right NOW.

Step One: Take your total weight in pounds and divide it by two to determine how much water you should drink per day. So if you weigh 200 pounds, you drink 100 ounces of water a day. It is best to spread your water intake throughout the day.
Your total body weight ______ ÷ 2 = ______ ounces of water you should drink per day.

Step Two: Drink 8 ounces every morning as soon as you wake up, preferably with vitamin D. Most people are deficient in vitamin D and taking vitamin D in the morning actually works to help people sleep better at night. Total body wellness includes hydration, nutrition, and sleep--why not tackle as many issues as you can first thing in the morning? This also helps start your day in a positive, motivational manner.

Step Three: Find a water bottle that sports your personality and lifestyle. Some people like big bottles and some like small, there are positives and negatives to both. The most important thing is you meet your daily intake goal. Pick a bottle that suits you.

Step Four: Did you have an intense workout today? Remember on days in which you have had a particularly difficult workout, it is not enough to hydrate with water. Drink plenty of water while exercising, and at least 20-24 ounces within the first hour post training. Serious athletes will also need to replace your lost electrolytes (lost through sweat). Choose an all-natural drink such as coconut water or a medical grade hydration drink such as Drip Drop on days that you have a workout that produces an intense dripping sweat.

Macronutrients are the three types of foods that we need to eat to survive: ***proteins, carbohydrates,*** and ***fats.***

You've probably gotten used to looking at nutrition labels to figure out how many calories are in a serving of whatever you're eating, right? On every packaged food item you buy, you have a nutrition label that will tell you how many calories, fats, carbohydrates, proteins, among a lot of other things such as vitamins, sodium, ingredients, etc., are contained in that food item. You need to be aware of what it is you're putting in your body.

Protein

The first macronutrient you should be concerned about eating is the most important for body composition, and that's PROTEIN. Simply, protein builds the body and keeps it functioning at optimal levels.

5 Reasons Why You Should Be Eating Protein:

1. **Muscle Protein Synthesis:** Muscle tissue is made up of proteins. When a person puts stress on a muscle, such as lifting weights, proteins become

damaged. Protein synthesis is the repairing of damaged proteins and replacing them with replicas of the original. The new muscle tissue is stronger and able to handle stress better than before. This is how muscle building works.

What's so great about muscle? Aside from being able to function better in life and looking great—adding muscle helps you lose fat. Muscle needs energy. A pound of muscle uses up to 150 calories a day, whereas a pound of fat only needs about 3 calories a day. Simply having a lot of muscle burns calories. Just remember—body fat does not need energy to maintain itself and muscle does, so you have to weight train in order to spark the protein synthesis.

What does this have to do with eating protein?

A moderate serving of high-quality protein maximally stimulates skeletal muscle protein synthesis in young and elderly subjects (Journal of the American Dietetic Association, 2009). According to a 2008 study in the American Society for Nutrition, ingesting just 20 g of dietary protein post workout is enough to maximize muscle protein synthesis after resistance exercise.

2. Thermic effect: Before I explain thermic effect, let us look at a different term—metabolism: the term commonly used to describe the process of breaking down food and turning it into energy. Most people have heard that in order to lose weight a person wants a high metabolism to burn off calories, right? This is true. But what raises your metabolism? Ironically, one of the best ways is eating. Food has what is called a thermic effect, which is the energy the body needs to eat, digest, and metabolize food. After you eat, your Basal Metabolic Rate (BMR) begins to rise. This rise can be fairly meager or it can be quite significant depending on how much you ate and the types of foods you ate. According to shapefit.com, fats generally raise your BMR by about 4%, carbohydrates by about 6%, and proteins by a whopping 30% --wow!

I have read other studies that suggest the thermic effect of protein is lower than the shapefit.com estimates, but everyone seems to agree that the thermic effect of protein is at least double that of your other macronutrients—carbs and fat.

In other words, eat more protein to burn more calories.

3. Increase in Glucagon: Consuming dietary protein increases the peptide hormone Glucagon. Glucagon raises concentrations of glucose in the bloodstream--it does the opposite of insulin—this leads to greater fat mobilization. Glucagon and insulin both help to regulate blood sugar. Basically, an increase in glucagon leads to greater fat loss during calorie restriction and less fat gain during overeating.

4. Cardiovascular Health: Multiple studies have shown that when people replace around 15% of their calories from carbohydrates with calories from protein, this lowers LDL cholesterol and triglycerides.

5. Satiety and Prevention of Weight Cycling Effect: A study found the fat loss success of many low carb diets had more to do with the increase in protein consumption than the reduction of carbohydrates. That study concluded that dietary protein was an effective treatment of obesity in that it improved metabolic function, increased satiety and energy levels, and decreased the weight cycling affect—the cyclical loss and gain of weight often referred to as yo-yo dieting.

Now. You're eating lots of protein. Where are you going to get your protein from?

Protein Sources

First, there are three main sources of protein -- animal, vegetable, and supplements.

Animal

Despite the myths purveyed by agents of the soy industry, by far the best source of protein is animal—MEAT. Eat meat! And plenty of it. Meat in its natural form (non-processed, organic, and steroid free) is one of the healthiest, nutritionally sound foods a person can eat. Animal meat is an excellent source of high quality protein.

So what kinds of animals should you be eating? Pretty much all of them. Birds, fish, eggs, cow, chicken, lamb, game...whatever you can think of. Just like you'll see with veggies, it is always a good idea to eat a wide variety of meat. Chicken might be a great source of lean protein; however, certain fish varieties will provide a better concentration of healthy saturated fats, beef will provide a quality source of iron and new amino acids, and eggs are loaded in nutrients that are not easily acquired in other food forms.

Non-Animal

Non-animal sources of protein such as soy products, beans, nuts, and other protein-dense veggies do provide protein; however, they are not ideal sources of optimal proteins. In order to get the five benefits of eating protein discussed above, you should be consuming probably about 30% of your daily caloric intake from protein and this would be very difficult to do on a non-meat diet.

Also animal meat, especially fish, is dense in Omega 3's—DHA, EPA, and ALA and you need all three. ALA you can get from plants. But non-meat eaters should be taking fish oil to get adequate amounts of DHA (over 30% of your brain is made up of this) and EPA (an important anti-inflammatory).

Flax seed oil cannot be your only source of Omega 3s because flax seed is only ALA and less than 5% can get converted into DHA. If you are a vegetarian, at least take microalgae oil. Vegetarians are typically deficient in Omega 3's.

Supplements

How can I get 20 grams of protein post workout quickly and easily? I don't have time to cook meat, I know I shouldn't eat processed meats; what is a busy person to do?

This is where supplements are useful and probably necessary. In the beginning of your new health and wellness journey, supplements shouldn't necessarily be a high priority; however, quality protein supplements can be an excellent way to meet your dietary protein demand – especially for the person with a busy lifestyle. In addition, supplemental protein like whey protein can provide you with powerful antioxidants, lower high blood pressure, and increase lean muscle mass.

How do I choose the right supplement?

I published this article http://strongfigure.com/kind-protein-buy/ to help people figure out what supplemental protein they should buy. These powders are my top picks based on

- Results
- Quality
- Taste
- Mixability
- Cost

And not necessarily in that same order. There are an abundance of protein powders available for purchase, all the way from plant proteins, and to egg and casein proteins. Choosing the best one can feel extremely overwhelming. You need to figure out what's most important to you.

What will you pay for?

- The best tasting powder?
- One that mixes well with smoothies and coffees and doesn't end up lumpy or chalky?

What do you value?

- Results over taste? Are you willing to choke down the fast-acting, muscle replenishing powder that does taste a bit chalky in order for optimal results?
- Is cost a limiting factor to you? Availability of purchase?
- What about ingredients? Do you want organic with no additives? Limited additives? Sweeteners?
- Do you need a powder that will help you recover from exercise or are you looking to add a nighttime chocolate shake to your routine?

Fortunately, since there are hundreds of protein powder options available to you, manufacturers are making so many blends and flavors that most of them don't taste too terribly awful. In fact, I don't mind the taste of most that I've tried; however, I'm also not picky. I've been given several tubs of protein from various friends because they couldn't stand the taste. (FYI--most of those proteins were plant-based powders).

We could spend hours discussing protein powders here, but the main goal I have for you is that if you can't get all your protein requirements from meat, dairy, eggs, etc., then it's not a bad idea to add a shake to your routine. Sample various types of powders and don't give up until you find something you truly enjoy. I promise, it's out there.

Blue River Health's BEST Protein Picks for a Healthier, Active, Well-Balanced Life:

Animal Sources (BEST PICKS):

- Beef
- Turkey
- Tilapia
- Lamb
- Salmon
- Cod
- Pork
- Shrimp
- Shellfish
- Chicken
- Eggs
- Cottage Cheese
- Greek Yogurt (plain has more protein and you can add

your own berries, etc., for taste)

Non Animal Sources (Ok picks):

- Beans
- Nuts
- Seeds
- Soy Products

Supplements (Good picks! Especially if weight training):

- Whey protein powders
- Casein protein powders
- Egg protein powders
- Plant-based protein powders

Circle your favorite items from the protein list. When you go to the store, buy these protein sources. Once you're home with plenty of protein, figure out how you want to eat your protein. Remember to try and divide up your grams of protein appropriately throughout the day. If you can aim for 20-30g of protein per meal and 10-15g per snack, that would be ideal.

Anything you can cook ahead of time, cook it and get it in your fridge for the week. You'll never have an excuse to be low on protein if you have 5 chicken breasts and two pounds of ground turkey already cooked, seasoned, and ready to be eaten. And if you keep items such as cottage cheese (which can also be blended with frozen berries if you don't like its texture), hard boiled eggs, and Greek yogurt in your fridge, snacking on high protein foods will become second nature.

When you go back to the store again, choose some different sources next time and experiment with different foods and recipes.

Fats

Fats sound like they would be bad for you; however, most fats are actually very good for you. These are the naturally occurring fats—saturated, unsaturated, polyunsaturated....they are all good (mostly).

So what is bad?

Food processing has created some bad fats called trans-fats. In an effort to make food last longer and feel softer in your mouth, food processors take regular unsaturated fats and hydrogenate them. This is bad. *Real bad.* In fact many health organizations refer to trans-fats as a contaminant byproduct of food processing. Trans-fats are edible but they have been linked to cardiovascular disease and obesity. Trans-fats are so bad that there are laws limiting them or banning them in other countries.

The United States has had proposals to ban trans-fats and in 2013 the United States Food and Drug Administration (FDA) officially said trans-fats are "generally not recognized as safe."

Have you heard that saturated fats are bad?

The dogma that fat, particularly saturated fat, is bad for you and carbohydrates are a better choice is likely the reason heart disease and obesity have both skyrocketed in the last 30-40 years. If you are wondering whether a fat is good or bad, simply ask yourself this: does this fat occur naturally? If the answer is yes, then by all means eat it. If the answer is no, then treat it like poison—it is.

Here are a few examples of good vs. bad fats:

- Coconut oil is natural, so it's good.
- Hydrogenated vegetable oil is not natural, so it's bad.
- Fat from beef is natural so it's good.
- Partially hydrogenated oils are not natural and very bad.

Think about it this way: early humans evolved from eating fats--particularly animal fats. The hunter-gatherer diet would have consisted of large amounts of fatty tissue. We were evolved to eat this stuff.

Most of those shelf oils you see in your baking aisle at the grocery store are bad—safflower, canola, vegetable oil—those oils that sit there in liquid form are usually hydrogenated and this makes them scary—stay away!

Healthy Fats

Most who are reading this have heard of essential fats or "healthy fats." Generally, these terms are referring to polyunsaturated and monounsaturated fats. But the truth is, it depends on the form the fat comes in. For example, safflower oil is a monounsaturated fat, one of the so called "healthy fats," but if the oil is hydrogenated to last on the store shelf, then the so-called healthy fat just became pretty unhealthy.

A good example of a monounsaturated fat is the avocado—those are very natural, so eat them. Nuts too! They grow on trees, not in laboratories.

A good example of a polyunsaturated fat is salmon—this fish comes from the sea so that is good.

Just remember: **Natural is good. Processed is bad.** I know this can be overwhelming for many people, so just remember to read your labels. A bottle of oil on a shelf will tell you if it's hydrogenated or partially hydrogenated. If it is, don't buy it! An avocado doesn't have a label. It's so natural that it doesn't even need one. Buy several. :)

Speaking of "good fats"—Omega 3s rock!

Omega 3s

The number one fat you absolutely do not want to limit is your Omega 3s—DHA, ELA, and ALA—these fats are the best. They are commonly found in fish. This is why one of the best things you can do for your health is to take fish oil.

Omega 3s and Omega 6s in Balance

Omega 6s (found in a lot of foods—nuts, soy, seeds, and most vegetable oils) are a little more controversial. And science is a bit all over the place on these cousins of the Omega 3s. The important thing is to balance your Omega 6s and Omega 3s.

Let's get back to the hunter-gatherer diet. The Paleo experts will tell you that the early hunter-gatherer had an Omega 6 to Omega 3 balance of 1:1; whereas, the average American today has a balance of 20:1. Wow! 20:1? What are we eating? Or better yet, what are we NOT eating?!?!

Chances are the average American is not eating enough fish, so when looking for healthy fats to add to your diet, don't forget to take fish oil.

Benefits of Fish Oil

- Fish oil consists of Omega 3's—DHA, EPA, and ALA and you need all three.
- ALA you can get from plants. But you should be taking fish oil to get adequate amounts of DHA (over 30% of your brain is made up of this) and EPA (an important anti-inflammatory).
- Flax seed oil cannot be your only source of Omega 3's because flax seed is only ALA and less than 5% can get converted into DHA.
- As stated in the protein section, if you are a vegetarian, at least take microalgae oil. Vegetarians are very deficient in Omega 3's.
- Children with high omega 3 intake were found to be 55% less likely to develop diabetes.
- Fish oil promotes weight loss.
- The anti-inflammatory effects of omega-3 fatty acids are thought to protect against atherosclerosis, the primary cause of heart disease.
- Omega 3s reduce leukotriene levels, and in turn help lessen the problems of people suffering with Inflammatory Bowel Disease.

- There have been numerous studies showing that fish oil reduces rates of cancer, stroke, and high blood pressure.
- As stated earlier, fish oil is GREAT FOR THE BRAIN, and it can also help with diseases such as Alzheimer's, Parkinson's, ADHD, Schizophrenia, Depression, and studies show that mother's consuming fish oil had children with higher IQ levels than mothers who were Omega 3 deficient.
- One study found that women who consumed fish oil were 70% less likely to develop breast cancer.

Important note:

Fish oil is great, but it oxidizes and can go bad really fast (which is normally a good sign that a food is good for you.) Consuming rancid fat is a big no-no: it acts as a mutagen, which could result in damage or impaired function of a particular gene and the accumulation of mutagens *could* lead to cancer. So keep your fish oil in a fridge and **take it with vitamin E**, which can reverse the oxidation.

Krill Oil as a Possible Replacement

Many believe krill oil may actually be a better alternative to regular fish oil because many of the mass producers of fish oil damage the product in production. The extraction process of krill oil is different and there is some evidence that it may be a better provider of Omega 3s due to this.

And some studies are suggesting that krill oil is absorbed within the body better.

No matter whether you choose fish oil or krill oil, just choose one and be sure to consume it each and every day. This will undoubtedly help your physical transformation, as well as your mood, brain power, and overall physical health.

Now. You're eating the appropriate amount of good fats. Where are you going to get your fat sources from?

Take a look at this list of these great, naturally occurring fat sources:

- Avocado
- Cold Pressed Organic Extra Virgin Coconut Oil
- Cold Pressed Organic Extra Virgin Olive Oil
- Nuts and seeds (Almonds, macadamia nuts, Brazil nuts, sunflower seeds, cashews...)
- Nut Butters (all natural peanut butter, almond butter, cashew butter...)
- Naturally occurring fats in animal products such as meats, eggs, cheeses...
- Butter or ghee (all natural, minimally processed)

When you go to the store, pick up some extra *natural* fat (meaning from animal sources or nuts/seeds). You don't have to buy a lot since it's very easy to consume a lot of fat in small quantities. You may want to pick up some coconut oil for cooking, baking (or for in your coffee!) Pick up an avocado or two to add to some of your meals, or grab some almonds to snack on. A great way to get a few fat grams into your diet is with a handful of mixed nuts. A little goes a long way, so you don't have to spend a fortune here.

Remember that you'll get some fat grams from your meat sources, depending which ones you choose. If you're a hungry person and you like to eat more food, choose leaner meat sources so that you can eat more meat and more fat, yet still be within your caloric goals (more on that to come). Chicken breasts and lean ground turkey are high in protein and low in fat, allowing you to meet your protein requirements while saving room for your favorite snack of almond butter and apples. On the opposite end, some of you may not care about nut butters and oils and you'd like to have a big juicy steak instead. Eat what makes you happiest and switch things up for variety and balanced nutrition as much as you can!

WARNING: Be cautious of hidden fats such as those in salad dressings, baked goods, or sauces and creams. A little is fine but too much can offset your fat allowance for the whole day! Besides, you want to try and eliminate as many processed foods from your diet anyway, so just limit these altogether!

Carbohydrates

The last, and possibly most misunderstood of all the macros: *What are carbohydrates?*

Your body uses carbohydrates to make glucose--the fuel that gives you energy and helps keep moving. Your body also uses glucose (sugar) and stores this in the liver and muscles for when energy is needed.

Carbs are frustrating because you need them; yet, if you eat too many of them you will store them. The key is going to be learning *what* foods are considered "carbs," *which* ones are the best carb sources to eat, and *when* is the best time of day to eat said carbs.

You can find carbs in the following food types:

- Fruits
- Vegetables
- Breads, cereals, and other grains
- Dairy, milk and sugar-sweetened milk products
- Foods containing added sugars (e.g., cakes, cookies, and beverages)

There are two main types of carbohydrates:

- Complex carbohydrates (what most people refer to as “good carbs”)
- Simple carbohydrates (what most people refer to as “bad carbs”)

The famous GOOD CARB vs. BAD CARB debate.

Everyone has heard of good carbs and bad carbs. Here's all you really need to know:

COMPLEX (GOOD) CARBS DIGEST SLOWLY, AND SIMPLE (BAD) CARBS DIGEST QUICKLY.

Complex (good) carbs:

- Green leafy veggies are always best when trying to eat a meal low in carbs.
- High fiber beans and veggies like brussel sprouts and lentils provide great carbs full of nutrients.
- "Whole wheat, whole grain, brown" (like whole wheat pasta or brown rice, quinoa and oats)
- Foods that have a low glycemic index rating

Simple (not-your-best-choices) carbs:

- Anything labeled "White" is a fast digesting carbohydrate (like white bread and white pasta and white rice)

- Pastries, cereals, most breakfast foods, most fruit yogurts, boxed dinners
- All desserts
- Most fruit and berries
- Food that has a high glycemic index rating.

So what's the importance of knowing the difference between a complex and a simple carb?

Easy: a complex carb choice is more nutritious than a simple carb choice. The only caveat to that is fruit. Fruit is nutritious—it just happens to convert to sugar rather quickly once eaten. Don't worry about that right now.

Some scientists have even been studying whether or not the high consumption of simple carbohydrates in the American diet is leading to health problems such as diabetes and heart disease. This is often why you hear carbs referred to as "good carbs" and "bad carbs."

All carbs break down into simple sugars once you eat them. It's just that simple carbs get broken down much faster and you feel hungry a lot sooner than if you ate complex carbs which contain fiber and keep you fuller, longer. That's why when you eat a piece of toast (white bread) or a piece of chocolate, you might get hungry again in 30 minutes, versus eating a serving of oats or black beans that will make you feel full for a while. The simple carb digests fast and makes you hungry again while the other more fibrous carb digests slowly and keeps you fuller, longer.

NOTE: Does that mean you should never eat a simple carb? No. This is all going to boil down to you and your goals. We're going to teach you how to consciously choose carbs that are the best for YOU at any stage of your revamp journey.

Here's a list of carbohydrate sources in a general order of most to least nutritious that will help you as you start making nutritional decisions within your new journey.

Healthy Carbohydrate Sources:

- Green leafy vegetables
- Other vegetables
- Berries
- Other fruits
- Nuts and seeds -- typically not thought of as a carbohydrate but many are fiber dense
- Beans and Peas
- Oatmeal
- Quinoa
- Brown rice
- Other grains

- Whole wheat breads and pastas (though for best results we recommend limiting quantities of these)

Fruit is Good, Vegetables are Better!

Let’s not forget that carbs--even though they can have such a bad reputation in the fitness industry--are good. They provide us with energy and we need them to survive. It’s the carbs that we choose to eat that will determine what kind of energy we run on--what’s the best, the most efficient fuel source? What makes us feel and look our best?

While fruit and many grains are full of vitamins, minerals, antioxidants, water, and fiber; what most people don't realize is that you can get the same vitamins and minerals from **vegetables**—vegetables that are not high in sugar, vegetables that will not spike your insulin (which causes your body to stop burning fat), and vegetables that are much lower in carbs and calories.

Vegetables are healthier, typically contain more overall nutrition, and will not leave you craving a sugary snack like other carb sources often do. And many veggies contain a high amount of water and fiber as well. When it comes to choosing between a donut and a grapefruit, of course choose the grapefruit. A croissant or steel-cut oats? Oats.

But whenever you can, fill your plate with veggies, as often as you can do so.

Just like all foods, when it comes to vegetables, variety is really important! Always try as many different veggies as possible. It's easy to pick a couple that are easy and familiar, but every vegetable is incredibly dense with a wide variety of nutrients; and it really is important to try new things, so why not start now? Here's our list of top veggies and their nutritional benefits. Which ones will you try? And why not try them all?!

Vegetables Health Benefits

- Kale: Anti-inflammatory, anti-oxidant, cancer preventative, and a source of at least four glucosinolates
- Spinach: Anti-inflammatory and anti-cancer from spinach phytonutrients--including more than a dozen flavonoids
- Broccoli: Digestive support, anti-cancer, cardiovascular support, and can enhance detoxification
- Sweet Potatoes: Blood sugar regulatory properties, anti-inflammatory, and antioxidants
- Peppers: Excellent source of carotenoids and loaded in vitamin C
- Turnip Greens: For total glucosinolate content, turnip greens outscore cabbage, kale, broccoli, and cauliflower. They have four times the calcium of cabbage--thus the bitter taste.
- Brussels Sprouts: A recent study shows daily consumption of Brussels sprouts improves stability of DNA inside of our white blood cells. And they are a cancer fighting powerhouse.

- Tomatoes: a recent study in Spain found that out of all commonly eaten foods, only the tomato and bell pepper contained vitamin C, vitamin E, and six of these carotenoids (alpha-carotene, beta-carotene, lycopene, lutein, cryptoxanthin and zeaxanthin).
- Garlic: Most Americans are sulfur deficient and garlic is perhaps the best source of sulfur. Garlic is also an excellent source of manganese, vitamin B6, and selenium.
- Onions: Sulfur rich, anti-inflammatory, cancer fighting, and one of the only quality sources of quercetin, a flavonoid antioxidant.
- Mustard Greens: Detox support, antioxidant rich, anti-inflammatory benefits, and they provide cardiovascular support
- Pumpkin/Squash: Squash has been noted for its blood-sugar regulatory benefits and they have unique antioxidants not found in other veggies.
- Lettuce (all types): One of the most underrated veggies on this list, eat a variety of lettuces to get quality antioxidants, folate, and vitamin K.
- Swiss Chard: Bone health, blood sugar benefits, and studies show chard prevents oxidative stress.
- Collard Greens: Digestive support, cardiovascular support, and an excellent source of vitamin K and omega 3 fatty acids.
- Beet Greens: Beet greens have a higher iron content than spinach and they contain 220% of the daily recommended value of vitamin A.
- Green/Red Cabbage: Eat both green and red cabbage for the variety of antioxidants and anti-cancer benefits.

- Celery: One of the best sources of phytonutrients, many of which are phenolic antioxidants. Great for your liver and digestive tract.
- Carrots: They are known for their carotenoids (beta-carotene) but a new Dutch study shows carrots might outperform green leafy veggies in protecting against cardiovascular disease. Carrots are also a top performer in a category of phytonutrients called polyacetylenes.
- Cauliflower: One of the leaders in antioxidants but perhaps more interestingly new research is looking at cauliflower's potential benefits in preventing the following inflammation-related health problems: Crohn's disease, inflammatory bowel disease, insulin resistance, irritable bowel syndrome, metabolic syndrome, obesity, rheumatoid arthritis, type 2 diabetes, and ulcerative colitis.
- Asparagus: Heart health, blood sugar regulation, digestive support, and anticancer properties.
- Seaweed: Helps with thyroid function, high in protein, and more calcium than broccoli. Also, a type of brown seaweed called kombu contains the pigment fucoxanthin, which may help your body metabolize fats for energy.
- Fennel: Unique phytonutrients; good for liver; plus helps cardiovascular and colon health.
- Leeks: Contains flavonoid kaempferol, which helps protect blood vessel linings from damage. Plus leeks contain important concentrations of B vitamin folate.
- Parsley: Studies have shown that parsley's volatile oils, such as myristicin, inhibit tumor formation in the lungs. It also helps protect against rheumatoid arthritis and promote heart health.
- Bok Choy: Cancer fighting, anti-inflammatory, and antioxidant rich -- another powerful cruciferous veggie.

- Dandelion Greens: Assists the immune system, helps with kidney health, and has cancer fighting properties.
- Radicchio: Improves digestion, improves cardiovascular health, anti-cancer properties, and a good source of vitamin K.
- Chives: Like onions and garlic, chives contain allicin, which lowers blood pressure and helps prevent heart disease.
- Endive: Helps detox and improve liver and gallbladder health. Also, helps in digestive health and heart health.
- Kohlrabi: Kohlrabi contains health-promoting phytochemicals such as isothiocyanates, sulforaphane, and indole-3-carbinol, which protect against prostate and colon cancers.
- Mushrooms: Immune system support, promotes cardiovascular health, contains antioxidants, and anti-inflammatory benefits.
- Zucchini: Promotes eye health and protects the colon from harmful chemicals known to cause cancer.
- Corn: Corn is underrated in its benefits. Corn contains a plethora of antioxidant phytonutrients, has blood sugar benefits, and aids in digestive health.
- Peas: Supports blood sugar regulation, protects against stomach cancer, and peas have anti-inflammatory benefits.
- Other veggies worth mentioning: cucumbers, escarole, eggplant, alfalfa sprouts, green beans, rutabaga, watercress.

More on Vegetables: Fresh vs. Frozen vs. Canned: Does it Matter?

Most people believe that fresh veggies are healthier over frozen or canned. If the vegetables are coming right out of said person's garden and being immediately eaten, then yes! It doesn't get much more nutrient-dense than that.

However, how often does this happen for the majority of most people?

FLASH FROZEN vegetables are awesome, and unless you get your veggies from a local, organic food source such as a farmer's market; you should probably buy the majority of your vegetables frozen. First, frozen vegetables are blanched (flash frozen) almost immediately once picked/chopped/diced. This preserves the bulk of the nutrients in the vegetable. Fresh vegetables have to be prepped, boxed, they travel for days, sit in the produce aisles until bought, then sit on your counters or fridge even longer...and all that time spent sitting, that vegetable is losing its nutritional value. Of course you can't really do this with all veggies—imagine trying to thaw Romaine for a salad. But you CAN choose frozen vegetables over fresh when you have the option.

"Once a perishable product is frozen at proper temperatures, it does not matter if the date expires because food kept frozen continuously is safe indefinitely. Products exposed to air can develop 'freezer burn' which does not affect the safety of the product, but can impact taste and quality." (Adapted information from PA Dept. Of Agriculture and American Frozen Food Institute)

As for canned? Most canned veggies are packed with other additives, and vegetables should not contain "additives." If you need to pick up canned vegetables, look for organic, low sodium versions of canned veggies if you can't get the vegetable frozen or fresh, first. Also, some stores carry BPA-free canned goods. If it's important to you in your quest to revamp your health to avoid BPA-free items, the can should contain a label or stamp letting you know if it's BPA-free or not.

Definitely limit canned fruits—especially the ones that contain added sugar.

Exceptions to canned veggies: canned/jarred sauerkraut, artichokes hearts, and diced tomatoes are very easy to buy in a can or jar. So if you buy these often, always try to buy organic whenever possible and read labels to make sure no sugar or artificial ingredients are added.

When to buy ORGANIC?

You don't have to buy organic all the time—it's expensive. You must understand though that your health shouldn't be a "luxury item" ; it's a necessity and worth a few more cents here and there.

Here's a basic "What to Buy Organic/What Not to Buy" list to help you choose safe foods and to avoid unnecessary toxins that can cause all sorts of free-radical damage to your cells.

Daily Green's Top Foods to buy ORGANIC:

- Meat
- Coffee
- Celery
- Peaches
- Strawberries
- Apples
- Blueberries
- Nectarines
- Bell Peppers
- Hot Peppers
- Spinach
- Kale
- Cherries
- Potatoes
- Grapes
- Summer Squash
- Tomatoes
- Cucumbers

Daily Green's Top Foods to SKIP Buying Organic:

- Onion
- Avocado
- Sweet Corn
- Pineapple
- Mango
- Asparagus
- Sweet Peas
- Kiwi
- Cabbage
- Eggplant
- Papaya
- Watermelon
- Broccoli
- Tomato
- Sweet Potatoes
- Mushrooms

- Grapefruit
- Cantaloupe

NEXT: Go shopping!

Circle your favorite carb sources from the lists above--as many as you want! Carbs are typically cheaper than proteins and fats, and a good variety of carbs--especially from vegetables--will ensure your nutrient intake is optimal. Want to be super awesome? Try two vegetables that you've never had before!

Buy your groceries--your proteins, your fats, and your carbs, and then pre-cook as much as you can for the week so that you have your food ready for you when you need to eat!

What if you really want some popcorn or a piece of dark chocolate? Treat yourself often to small servings of the foods that make you happy. Completely avoiding or trying to eliminate these foods may trigger binge eating behaviors and that is NOT healthy.

If you think you have a serious sugar addiction (sugar does in fact act like a drug with addictive properties) there is one way to overcome your sugar high. Try slowly decreasing your sugar intake day-by-day. When you have successfully decreased your intake to bare minimal levels, try avoiding all sugar for about 28-30 days. Research shows that anyone who can avoid sugar for about one month will no longer get the intense cravings and won't feel tied to eating it.

Eat fruit and berries to combat the sweet tooth and have small desserts when celebrating special occasions. Don't cut out desserts from your life forever—just be aware of the potential side-effects of too much sugar in the body and how to eat wisely.

How to Avoid Eating Added Sugars

1. Always choose water over sugar-sweetened sodas and juices.
2. If you must drink juice, find one made from 100% fruit juice and then dilute it with water.
3. Breakfast cereals (which are mostly simple sugars or have sugars added) are one of the worst sugary foods that we don't normally think about. Look for ones that contain 4 grams or less of sugar.

Carbs come in all sizes and shapes. In the end--they are made up of sugar. It's up to you--and always will be--to decide which ones you will choose for your body. Look for these ingredients in the nutrition label. (I know it will take a while to remember all this information. However, if you see any ingredient that ends in "ose," it's an added sugar. Beware!)

The following is a list of "added sugars." Just do your best avoid these products *as much as possible*. They are toxic carbs!

- Brown Rice Syrup
- Brown Sugar
- Cane Juice
- Corn Sweetener
- Corn Syrup
- Dextrose
- Fructose
- Fruit Juice Concentrates
- Glucose
- High Fructose Corn Syrup
- Honey
- Invert Sugar
- Maltose
- Malt Syrup
- Molasses
- Raw sugar
- Sucrose

Though a little bite of chocolate here and there isn't going to kill anyone, there are dangers in eating *too much* sugar.

> *"Sugar is a drug that has no nutritional value and is an addictive chemical."* Evita Ochel, Author and Holistic Nutritionist

Sugar may:

- Stop the brain from producing serotonin resulting in mood swings, unhappiness, irritability and other negative symptoms.
- Cause teeth to deteriorate, cause cavities in the teeth, cause gums to bleed, and even cause one to lose teeth.
- Make the pancreas overwork in its production of insulin leading to insulin resistance and type 2 diabetes. And type 2 diabetes is now being linked to Alzheimer disease.
- Clog arteries, cause hypertension (high blood pressure, weaken arteries, cause strokes and heart attacks.
- Increase the risk for osteoporosis.

Sugar is also responsible for the following:

- Stripping valuable nutrients from the body.
- Making your immune system slow down to a crawl.
- Paralyzing the white blood cells responsible for squashing invaders like viruses and bacteria for up to around 5 hours and reduces their ability to work properly by up to 40%.
- It elevates cortisol in the body which causes increases to various infections as well as general organ malfunction, including heart disease.
- It causes damage to literally every system or organ in our body, including the liver and kidneys.
- It's linked to learning disorders in kids such as ADD/ADHD.
- Sugar is directly related to cancer: the higher the sugar consumption, the greater the risk of cancers.

Processed Foods Contain Sugar!

Beware of hidden sugars in processed food--this is why so many health-conscious individuals try to avoid foods that are processed (altered by man) and that's because too many unhealthy substances, like sugar, are added to the foods. Many packaged or processed foods contain high levels of hidden sugar. They may be easy to prepare and fill your family up for cheap, but too much sugar causes rapid swings in energy and blood sugar, and can contribute to many serious health problems--all listed above.

Common foods (you might not realize) that contain added sugars:

- Instant Mashed Potatoes
- White Bread and Pasta
- Canned Soups and Vegetables
- Cereals
- Low-Fat Foods (Many foods labeled low fat have been stripped of its natural--typically good--fat and the fat has been replaced with sugar!)

LESSER KNOWN FACT OF THE DAY:

Q. What happens when there is too much sugar in your bloodstream?

A. "It starts attacking your skin. All that sugar attaches to those protein molecules, collagen and elastin. And it turns those beautiful, supple skin cells into these firm, rigid things causing sagging, wrinkling, everything we don't want on our face."-- Brooke Alpert, co-author of The Sugar Detox: Lose Weight, Feel Great, and Look Years Younger.

Satisfy your sweet tooth with naturally sweet food such as fruit, peppers, and sweet potatoes.

Obviously, overeating sugar is a terrible idea. Have a cupcake on your birthday or your favorite candy on Halloween. There is a true balance to living life healthy and happy—and that includes your sanity too! *Balance is healthy*. When you are able to balance the treats with a healthy lifestyle made up of great food choices and plenty of exercise, you'll find that those treats that once took over your life, may just be a thing of the past. So start getting into the habit of being mindful of your food choices and knowing when it's ok to have that treat--without going overboard.

One last thing on Macronutrients:

A question that tends to pop up a lot is, "How do I know if a food item is a protein, a carb, or a fat?"

When you read a label--let's take peanut butter for example--you can see that peanut butter contains 7g protein, 8g carbs, and 16g fats. Seven grams is a decent amount of protein in only a couple of small spoonfuls, so many people actually think that peanut butter is a high "protein food." But let's look at that label again. Of the three macronutrients--proteins, fats, and carbs--which one has the highest number beside it? That's right, fat. Peanut butter contains 16g of fat which is more than double the

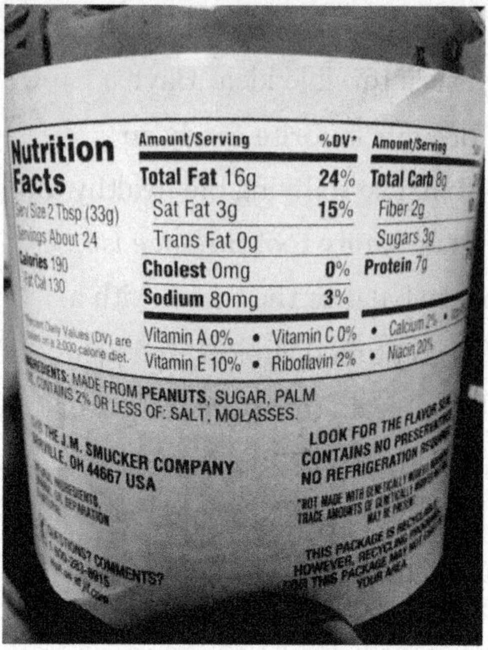

protein and exactly double that of carbs. So this is a great example of a "good fat" food (if you bought the all-natural kind...and technically, almond butter is even healthier).

Figuring out a protein food, a fat food, or a carb food is so easy! All you have to do is look at the label. If you're trying to consume a food high in protein, peanut butter isn't your best option. (Yes, your body still uses the 7g of protein found in the peanut butter, but your body will process this food as a FAT. Meaning, you will digest it slowly, it will keep you fuller for longer, and the protein is just an added bonus.) Don't let this upset you. **Peanut butter is a good fat that contains a little bit of protein.** When you eat it, your body says, *"Yummm!! Look at this healthy monounsaturated fat she needs for energy, satiety, and to protect her vital organs! Oh, and look at those couple grams of protein too! Let's toss that in with her energy needs."*

In other words, when you're trying to add protein to your diet, don't choose a food that is higher in fat than it is in protein. And don't choose a food that is higher in carbs than it is protein--if you're trying to eat a high-protein food. It may sound confusing at first, but start paying attention to labels now. The more you read them, the more food will start making sense to you!

Let's look at chicken breast for example. You'll get 24 grams of protein and 2 grams of fat from a chicken breast. Yes, you get a couple fat grams from chicken, but it's a protein source. That's how you tell the difference.

Let's look at four ounces of 93/7 ground turkey.

- One serving size of 4 oz cooked ground turkey contains 120 calories
- In 4 ounces of lean turkey, one will consume 0 grams of carbs, 2 grams of fat, and 28 grams of protein

This turkey counts as:

A) A carb
B) A fat
C) A protein

You're right. It's definitely a protein. A whopping 28 grams at that! So if you need a meal high in protein, eat the turkey or the chicken, not the peanut butter.

So now you know: proteins, fats, and carbohydrates are the necessary macronutrients needed to sustain life.

While ***macro*****nutrients** make up your daily calories, we also need several ***micro*****nutrients** to truly optimize our health and well-being. What are **Micronutrients?** Your vitamins and minerals that work to regulate your body processes.

MICRO-nutrients.

Micronutrients are important when it comes to how you choose your foods, or simply, your nutrient optimization. Let's look at this scenario. Tom is a 170 lb guy who works out three to four times a week and eats roughly 2000 calories a day. All good so far, right? Except that most of Tom's food choices aren't the best for optimizing his nutrition. If Tom chooses to have a donut for breakfast, a couple slices of pizza for lunch, a bowl of pasta for dinner with a side of garlic bread--he's likely hitting at least 800 calories worth of simple carbs here--not to mention his smoothie that has fruit in it, the piece of chocolate he found in his desk, and the small bowl of popcorn he had before bed....you get where I'm going. He can eat these things--anyone can eat these things--but how will he feel? How would you feel if this was (or is?) your typical diet? What do you think Tom's energy is like? What is his digestive system like? Where's his fiber? His protein? His good fats? How are his insides functioning?

By the way, this was similar to my lifestyle while in college, minus the workouts and add in too much Chinese Food. I was an English major who knew nothing about health. I gained over 40 pounds in my four years of late-night unnecessary carb loading, my digestive system was shot, I had constant bladder issues from dehydration, my skin was pale and blotchy, and I just wasn't healthy. I had to learn everything for myself the hard way. This book isn't just me telling you, "this is what you need to do to be healthy" ; I'm showing you that if I can do it, you can do it too. You're in a place where I've been, and I know that it's possible to change. This is my way of helping.

So what if Tom ate a breakfast that included a veggie-based omelet instead of a donut or a bowl of sugary cereal? What if his lunch was a taco salad over mixed greens with brown rice and black beans? What if he had an apple for his snack instead of the chocolate? What if he had spaghetti squash pasta with a side of asparagus over a grilled salmon filet for dinner? And what if his bedtime snack was a smoothie bowl with frozen berries, chopped kale, protein, and some homemade granola sprinkled on top?

Compare Tom's energy now, to the "other" Tom. His calories are the same. He's eating at the same times. He's not dieting down. His organs are functioning at a higher rate. His digestive system works properly because his carb sources contain fiber. His energy is outstanding, and all due to the types of foods he has chosen to eat.

That's what you have to do when you eat. You need energy and fiber. You need to build and maintain muscle mass, and you need to protect your bones and organs. You need healthy insides. You need to fight disease. You need to be well. Where are Tom's *MICRO*nutrients in the first scenario? How many vitamins and minerals is Tom getting from pizza, donuts, popcorn, and pasta? And what about the other food plan? Which plan contains more life-sustaining quality nutrients?

How are YOU going to optimize your calories?

Eating pizza, popcorn, donuts, and pasta is fun and it has its place in our food culture. I'll never tell you that you have to cut them out. I will say that it's probably not the best idea to eat these foods every single day. If you can learn to choose foods based on their *micronutrient value* and then splurge only *every now and then* on the pasta and pizza, you'll see a tremendous change in not just your physical appearance but your mood, energy, skin, and overall health.

When you know how to optimize your calories, eat what you need to for your daily energy expenditure, and how to have a treat when you want one, you won't only get your desired results, but you will be on your way to living a smarter, happier, healthier, well-balanced life. Most of your vitamins and minerals should come from food, and you only need a supplement when your food intake is not providing sufficient sources. This is just one of the many benefits of eating a wide variety of macronutrients.

But the hard part for so many of us--and perhaps one of the questions that has lead you to this book is, *"How do I figure out what and how much to eat?"*

Understanding FOOD and YOU

Eating a wide variety of macronutrients while aiming for the best *micro*nutrient choices will lead you to the best shape of your life. And knowing your macronutrient profile benefits both your physical AND mental health—especially if you've dieted for too long and your perception of food has been damaged.

What's a macro-profile?

The amount of calories consumed by any individual is immensely important. You now understand what macro- and micronutrients are, and combining this knowledge with the understanding of how much protein, carbohydrates, and fats you need to eat on any given day, is the ultimate key for long term success, as well as for great body composition...meaning, what makes you look good!

At this point you might be thinking, *"Yes! I want to know how much to eat!"* Or you may be thinking, *"No! I don't want to worry about calories. I just want to eat what I want and be healthy!"*

Guess what? You can have both. No person should have to sit around and count calories for the bulk of one's lifetime just to be able to "stay fit and healthy." Counting, logging, and tracking can be obsessive and can lead to potential eating disorders.

And guess what else? Every single person is different. You metabolize food differently than I do and vice versa. Even two people of the same height and weight who eat the exact same foods and perform the exact same workout will metabolize food differently. Why? We're just all too different.

So how do you figure out what to do?

In my experience, the more you dive into nutrition, the more complicated it can get. In order to remove as much confusion as possible, I want to present you with what I believe are the three best methods of eating for wellness (and weight loss).

Why three? Like I said before, we're all very different human beings. Some of you love accuracy and numbers. Some of you like balance and flexibility. Some may enjoy knowing exactly what to eat without thinking much about it. And some of you may be a combo of all of these. And because you and I are going to metabolize food differently, react to foods differently, and enjoy foods differently, you'll have to figure out what is going to work best for you--long term. That's what makes this healthy: you can change, long term, for the better, and live much healthier and happier.

I think it's safe to say that most of us know by now that diets don't work. Even if they work for a while, none of them should be followed long term, and some may even cause significant metabolic damage (meaning, you'll have an even harder time losing weight the more you try). We all need to live a healthy lifestyle supported by nutrient dense foods and foods that also make us happy.

And once you know what your body needs on a day-to-day basis, making healthy food choices becomes as natural as riding a bike. You may take a while to learn, you may even fall off a couple times and be scared to get back on. But in the end? You'll learn successful habits that will carry you where you need to go in life.

Some people just like being told what to eat and when. And while I could sit down and talk with you individually to help you figure this out, it's not necessarily what this book is about. I don't do 30-day fixes that leave you binging on ice cream on the 31st day, or advise someone to eat under 50g of carbs every day. This isn't a quick fix book--it's a lifestyle changing, good-habit forming book. I know we live in a society that craves instant fixes, but your body will never be a quick-fix. Why not try a few more long-term methods and discover how you can best live your own healthiest life?

If you DO however want to sit down for one-on-one coaching, please contact me here for individual health coaching or at blueriverhealth.com.

Option One: Try out PALEO.

Odds are, you may have heard of the "Paleo Diet." And it does kind of sound like a popular fad. However, I don't want you to think of this way of eating like a "diet" a "fad" or anything else with a negative connotation. You can Google "Paleo" and get more information than I can provide here (there are already several different books about just the Paleo way of eating). However, I can give you the simple, healthy version that will help you the most--if this turns out to be a good fit for you.

How do you know if the Paleo way of eating is right for you?

- You hate counting calories and tracking food
- You love eating the good fats, including animal fats (think nuts, avocado, steak, pork/bacon, almond butter...)
- You could give up sugar and sweets and processed foods fairly easily
- You have at least 50+ pounds to lose and you want to start losing NOW
- You aren't very active (at least not yet)
- You like to eat "real" food
- You enjoy cooking meat and you like to experiment with recipes

- You're pretty disciplined when it comes to eating out or going to social events

How to eat the Paleo way:

- The Paleo method is often called the caveman method. If a caveman had access to it, you can eat it. That means food in its purest form--before man touches it.
- No, that doesn't mean you have to kill your own wildlife for a bit of protein and it doesn't mean that you have to eat all foods raw either. You're just trying to eat naturally wholesome foods.
- Eat a lot of veggies--any of them.
- Eat meat, fish, eggs, wild game, store-bought meat (preferably grass-fed, free range meats)
- Eat berries, nuts, seeds, and some fruit (don't go overboard on fruit--it's a lot of sugar--but don't cut it out completely. Two servings per day is generally enough.)
- Typically all legumes (beans, peanuts, lentils), as well as most grains (oats, rice, breads, wheat, quinoa), are a no-no for strict Paleo eaters. I say, if you're used to buying boxed and frozen dinners and ordering Chinese take-out, then some high fiber beans, some quinoa (a high-protein grain), and a handful of peanuts every now and then will be fine. This is my opinion though. Some Paleo eaters will go as far as avoiding potatoes. I say a life without sweet potatoes is a sad one. And dairy? Forget it. Again--I say this should be up to you. There are a host of pros and cons when it comes to dairy and in my opinion, a bowl of cottage cheese shouldn't be outlawed. I mean, some cavemen had to have had goats they milked, right? Take the "no-nos" of a Paleo diet with a grain of salt. If you want to be strict for faster results, go for it. If you're in the process of switching from frozen pizza to learning what quinoa and kefir are (kefir is

a high protein and good gut-bacteria dairy product) then by all means, treat this as a learning process. I suppose some people would say, "What's the difference between a Paleo and a whole foods diet?" And really, not much. It all depends on how strict you want to be with your selections. Protein (meats and eggs), vegetables, berries, and good fats are a typical Paleo diet. Adding in some whole grains, organic dairy, and a few potatoes shouldn't harm your dieting efforts if you want them. I hope this wasn't confusing!

- Another side story: There was a time in my life that I ate Paleo so strictly that I gave up beans, fruit, dairy, sweet potatoes, oats, quinoa, you name it. I ate vegetables, meat, almonds...and that might've been it. In the long run--it lead to emotional distress and some binged carb eating. It just wasn't best for *me* even though I know so many who truly love it. So I say if you're going to try a Paleo diet, here's the BEST advice I can give you: **if it once swam, flew, walked, breathed, or grew out of the ground, it's ok to eat.** Eat REAL food and the less processed, the better. This plan works well -- especially for those eager to drop fat, and fast!
- And seriously, if you need a dark chocolate square every now and then, don't deprive yourself. Work hard, every day, but do NOT get into a restriction mindset. Eat healthy, whole, and real foods. When your office is eating donuts, do not feel deprived, make the conscious choice to feel uncomfortable for a few moments, walk away, and continue working. And when you truly feel that your body is craving a little sweet treat or a salty snack, it's ok. You have the power to make the choice: eat it and hop RIGHT back on the Paleo wagon, or opt for some fruit or salted nuts instead. You can do what you set your mind to as long as you have persistence and patience, coupled with the ability to cut yourself some slack every so often if or when you

take a misstep. Like anything, you can strive for perfection but it's ok to make mistakes along the way!

Bonus Tips:

- You can Google and Pinterest the sh** out of some Paleo recipes. My favorite Paleo website is paleomg.com.
- Don't get side-swept by all the "Paleo desserts" you'll find (and trust me, people will turn anything they can into a Paleo dish). A Paleo dessert means that someone made a donut out of all paleo ingredients: coconut or almond flour, organic molasses, organic butter, etc.....however you make donuts. Paleo desserts are really good...just not eaten in excess. If you're going to substitute the apple fritter for a Paleo cookie, go for it! If you're going to eat an entire batch of Paleo cookies "because it's Paleo," you're not doing anything for your health.
- For some reason, bacon is synonymous with Paleo. Bacon is a wonderful food. A pack or two of bacon per day will leave you thirsty as hell and with way too many calories and fat grams and sodium consumed. Just like anything--moderation is key.
- Eat veggies--as much as you want. Protein--roughly 20-30g per meal. Eat nuts, seeds, fruit, and berries in small amounts. Have a sweet potato, black beans, oats or quinoa if and when you need it. Avoid dairy if you're intolerant, but if not, cottage cheese is high in protein and though not necessarily "Paleo," it's a healthy form of dairy that mixes well with a lot of other foods like nuts and berries. And have a treat only when you need one.
- The stricter you are, the faster you'll lose weight. Eat "clean." The Paleo diet is not a low calorie one, but it's pretty darned effective at fat burning if you give it your best shot--especially if you have a lot of weight to lose.

Option Two: Count Your Macros:

Macro eating means you know exactly how many grams of carbs, proteins, and fats that YOU need to eat each day in order to be successful, lose weight (if that's your goal), have energy, and sustain a healthy lifestyle method of eating. I love macro counting because it's just so clear cut. A macro eating plan would be great for

- People who love numbers
- Those who like tracking foods and progress
- Those who love knowing and understanding what's going into the body--reading labels and figuring out what makes up the composition of each food
- Those who want to know exactly how much to eat and that's it--nothing more, nothing less
- Those who are good at following direction
- Those who like eating a variety of different foods
- Those who wants to save a little room for dessert every now and then
- Those who are disciplined in habit, but not so much in food choice or social events

How to track your macros:

This is the golden ticket for macro counters: the great and amazing macro formula!

Figure out your proper macronutrient profile:

1. What's your activity level? (Most people will be 11-13)

- 11: Sedentary. None or extremely little physical activity. You might be in grad school, injured, etc. You don't exercise (much if at all) and your job is sedentary.
- 12: You work out 3-5 hours a week. All who do just cardio (no weight training) will fall into this category.
- 13: You train 5-10 hours per week. You lift heavy weights and do interval conditioning workouts. Bodybuilders, Powerlifters, Strongman/woman training, CrossFitters.
- 14: You train 10-15 hours per week. Same type of lifting as above.
- 15: You train 15-20 hours per week, same as above, sometimes more than once a day.
- 16: You're a professional athlete

So what did you determine to be your activity level?

____

Whatever your activity level, add a ".5" if your job is active and you stay on your feet most of the day.

What is your new activity level number now?

____

2. Multiply your current weight (in pounds) by your activity level:

__________x___________=___________

Body weight in pounds x Activity level = Total Calorie Goal

This product is your total calorie goal for a healthy functioning metabolism.

3. Now take your weight in pounds and divide it by 2.2:

_________/2.2=___________

This is your daily recommended allowance of fat grams.

4. Take your fat gram allowance and multiply it by 2:

_______ x _______ = ________

This is your daily grams of protein goal.

5. To get your carbs, multiply your fat grams by 9: ______x 9 = __________. Then multiply your protein grams by 4: ______ x 4 = ___________.

Add these two numbers together: ______ + ______ =

____

Subtract this number from your total daily calories in number 2: ______ - _____ = ______

Divide this number by 4: ______/4 = _______

This is your daily recommended grams of carbs.

6. List your numbers:

________ Total calories

________ Fat grams

________ Protein grams

________ Carb grams (25-30 grams of fiber each day should come from appropriate carb sources. ← Don't forget this!)

Where things get complicated:

In my experience, people are either overeating or undereating, and nine times out of ten, they're under-eating protein and overeating carbs and fat.

Some people are just under-eating everything because they're scared to eat too much!

If you see your numbers above and you are thinking to yourself, "I'll never hit these numbers, that's too low or too high," that's ok! I don't want you to hit these numbers tomorrow.

How to get to the right numbers:

Unless you have already been tracking your calories, you probably don't know how many calories you're currently eating. And the numbers you listed above are maintenance numbers for your current weight. But what if you're supposed to be eating 1800 calories, and yet for months you've been eating 1400? Or what if you're supposed to be eating 1600 but you've been eating 2300?

This is important. You've got to get your metabolism functioning optimally before you can do anything else. How?

1. Track your calories for a week and see what you typically eat.

2. Very slowly, start adding or subtracting calories (no more or less than 100-150 per week) until you reach your target number.

3. When you hit your calorie goal that you calculated, aim for getting these calories met every day for at least a week. Don't worry about the other numbers--just calories.

4. When you can successfully hit your calories for a week, then focus on hitting calories AND protein for a week.

5. Once you can successfully hit these numbers for a minimum of a week, then start aiming for all your macros: calories, protein, fats, and carbs.

6. Calories and protein are the two most important numbers. You can fudge the other two slightly--sometimes you may want more carbs on a workout day and other days, not so much. As long as you stick to your calories and protein, you should be ok!

7. Don't forget fiber and water. 5 ounces of water per every 100 calories you eat and 25-30 grams of fiber a day.

8. Stay at the numbers you calculated for a minimum of two weeks, preferably a month, and keep track of your energy, mood, and appetite. Weigh yourself a couple times a week. Your weight should stabilize. This is how we know your metabolism is functioning properly ***and then you can move on.***

What do I do after I hit maintenance for a few weeks?

When you hit the right macro numbers and you stay there for a bare minimum of two weeks you can start doing whatever you want! (Well, sort of.) You really have about four options:

A. You can "cut" your calories by about 10% if your goals are fat loss. Cut SLOWLY though because if you cut too quickly you'll just screw up your metabolism and have to start this process all over again!

B. You can "reverse diet" to add strength and muscle. If your goal is get really strong and lean, start adding 10% to your diet each week while you slowly get stronger and put on some good solid muscle. Make sure you're lifting HEAVY or it's not going to be muscle you're adding to your frame. Cut back later once you've met your strength goals--and cut slowly to preserve your strength. Since this book is designed for beginners learning about general health and wellness, I wouldn't choose this option unless you're already weightlifting.

(For clarification purposes, "HEAVY" lifting means lifting in sets less than 8-12 reps and the weight should be so challenging to you that it feels damn near impossible to finish your last 1-3 reps.)

C. You can stay where you are and add intensity to your workouts--IF you're already working out. If you aren't working out yet, definitely add weightlifting and walking to your routine before cutting any calories. If you're already lifting, try adding more HIIT (high intensity interval training) to the end of your workouts. I wouldn't add anything more than 6-12 minutes, and really get your heart-rate up when doing so. Don't cut any calories until you've tried or are ready to try these options. If you're a beginner to exercising--no worries! We've got all the info you need to get started with fitness, coming up.

**See our section on HIIT/Interval Training in the next chapter!*

D. Stay where you are! The majority of you are here to learn how to eat healthier and live a more fit and active lifestyle. Once you know your maintenance calories, work on learning how to hit them daily without using scales and calorie trackers so that you can turn your healthy living into a lifestyle--not a fitness-tracking program that you get tired of.

The caveat to macro counting: even though this method seems pretty precise, you've got to keep in mind how different we all are, how uniquely our bodies work, and how "off" calories may sometimes be. It's actually common for a nutrition label to be "off" by several calories per serving. And factors such as previous dieting history, genetics, age, etc., can determine how many calories your body will actually burn. Eating a handful of almonds will burn more calories metabolically than it would if you ate the same amount of calories in almond butter. You'd also absorb less fat from the almonds than the butter (you have to do more work to eat the almonds than the butter). So keep all this in mind. Numbers are AWESOME but they're never going to be "exact."

Some of the newest research is showing that calorie counting is a bit more imprecise than nutritionists originally thought.

- You may log an apple on your calorie-counting app that says 83 calories when really, the apple was 118.
- One large sweet potato can have up to a 500 calorie difference when just logging "large sweet potato."

- Some nutritionists may argue that if you log your food in grams, your calories will be more precise. True. If I log 100g of a sweet potato, I might get a more accurate calorie number than just logging "large sweet potato." But who's setting the database for the gram conversion? And how do you know how exactly your body processes the sweet potato?
- Food companies use up to five different methods to label calorie counts on their foods--the FDA permitting them to be up to 20% *inaccurate* in either direction. If a label says 150 calories, what that really means is that you may be eating anywhere between 130-180 calories.
- This is going to shock you -- but you don't actually absorb all the calories you consume. Some calories actually pass through us undigested and this differs from food to food. You're looking at an average of a 10% error on your calorie absorption from food.
- How you prepare/chop/blend your food can change the overall calorie absorption and you can actually average a 90% error in calorie absorption from just preparing and cooking!
- You are different from every other person. Your own unique gut bacteria will absorb calories differently from others.
- People suck at eyeballing portions--which is why if you're going to macro-count, you've got to use a scale. One tablespoon of almond butter is shockingly small. Tell that to someone who counts a TBS as getting the largest spoonful of almond butter she can on a spoon and she'll be one sad little puppy. She could be "off" by over 100 calories with that spoonful!

As hard as it really is to understand your body and how much food it really is absorbing, some people truly enjoy the process of logging, tracking, and counting. If you realize that you could be off by a good 25% at the end of the day and you're ok with this, by all means track! For some people, it's just easy (and fun!) to see what you're eating, when you're eating it, and even though there is room for error, you have a database in front of you telling you what you're eating and will allow you make tweaks when needed. This is the format I choose just for the fact that I know I'm in a ballpark number each day. I'd rather be close than completely off base. BUT, if you're not a tracking and logging type of person and you think it seems pointless when the numbers can be so "off," try the next method.

Option Three: Use Your Body: More specifically, your fist and your brain.

Harping on the last statement of numbers never quite being "exact," this is the eating method designed on helping you eat the right amount of food *without* tracking calories each day. It's a little riskier of a method that will require a bit of trial and error, but those of you who don't like keeping track of every calorie will love this.

The palm method is adopted from Dr. John Berardi's Precision Nutrition program and it's FANTASTIC for

- Those who want as close to an accurate caloric guideline as possible--without counting any calories.
- Those who understand that portion sizes play a much bigger role in weight loss and gain than most adhere to.
- Those who want to eat a wide variety of whole foods without necessarily having to do a lot of food-planning.
- Those who want the simplest method of healthy eating.

Some people are going to LOVE this. If this is you, you understand that tracking can be "off" and you'd rather just eat the right foods in appropriate portions in accordance to what your body needs. How do you eat healthy without tracking anything?

Use your palm.

1. Your palm is proportionate to YOU. It's an ideal tool for food measuring.
2. 1 palm = 1 protein serving.
3. 1 whole fist = 1 veggie serving.
4. 1 cupped handful = 1 carbohydrate serving.
5. 1 thumb size = 1 healthy fat serving.

Now put this method into place.

For women:

Each meal should contain

- 1 palm of protein
- 1 fist of veggies
- 1 cupped handful of carbs
- 1 thumb of fat

3-4 meals will provide 1200-1500 calories. Adjust to add more meals as needed to meet calorie goals. No one should eat less than 3 meals per day.

Active women typically do well with 4-6 servings of each of the macronutrient food groups each day.

For men:

Each meal should contain

- 2 palms of protein
- 2 fists of veggies
- 2 cupped handfuls of carbs
- 2 thumbs of fat

3-4 meals will provide 2300-3000 calories. Adjust or remove portion sizes as needed to meet calorie goals. No one should eat less than 3 meals per day--even if you have to adjust portion sizes.

Active men typically do well with 6-8 servings of each of the macronutrient food groups each day.

How to Adjust Portions:

You may need less food if you:

- Are trying to lose weight
- Aren't getting the results you want
- Are not very active
- Feel too full after eating
- Are smaller for your size
- Eat frequently throughout the day

What you need to do:

- Women: Remove ½ cupped handful of carbs and/or ½ thumb of fat from a few meals each day.
- Men: Remove 1 handful of carbs and/or 1 thumb of fat for a few meals each day.

You may need more food if you:

- Aren't gaining the muscle you're after (must be currently weightlifting)
- Are trying to gain muscle
- Feel hungry/not satisfied after meals (you may be experiencing an "adjustment period" if you're currently over-eating)
- Eat less frequently during the day
- Larger for your size
- Are very active throughout the day

What you need to do:

Women: Add ½ cupped handful of carbs and/or ½ thumb of fat to a few of your meals each day.

Men: Add 1 cupped handful of carbs and/or 1 thumb of fat to a few of your meals each day.

Always pay close attention to your food portions, your results, and adjust as needed. Even though this system seems simple--and it is--if you just start grabbing things after a while without fully paying attention to sizes, you could end up overeating.

But what about dairy?

Not everyone eats or even needs dairy, but some people are big fans. If you enjoy dairy, read the label. If you want cottage cheese, it's typically higher in protein than fats and carbs. It can be your protein source for ONE meal. If you like a cheese that's higher in fat? Count it as your thumb of fat. Just read labels and I wouldn't have more than 1-2 dairy servings per day.

Congratulations! You're learning how to eat better and you've even stepped up the water drinking. Now? Let's get moving.

DISCLAIMER:

If you have battled any type of eating disorder and tend to become obsessive when keeping track of food, it's good to know this about yourself and to understand that there's nothing wrong with wanting to keep things simple. Choose option one (the Paleo Method) or option three (the palm method) and just do your very best to make smart food decisions when you eat.

If the thought of choosing a method that's going to work best for you stresses you out, or you're not quite confident in yourself to start making these important adjustments to your diet, please visit us at:

http://blueriverhealthandwellness.com/coaching

We'd love to help you personally figure this out and we will work with you to find a coaching package that best suits your needs.

In this chapter you'll learn the basics for becoming more active. Don't worry. We're not going to make you buy gym memberships or sign up for marathons (unless you want to). We just want to show you how easy--and ESSENTIAL--it is for your health to be a more active person.

What you do and how much of it you do is going to be up to you. Again, being active for a combined total of 60 minutes per day is the ultimate goal.

So let's get started! How fit are you already, and where/how do you start exercising for better health?

For many people, the thought of going to the gym leaves them feeling nauseous. "Why go to the gym when all the people there are already in amazing shape and will judge me?"

To start moving more, you don't need to join a gym right away. All you need is the motivation (your "WHY") and the ability to get up and move. Every fitness expert will tell you to start small. Walk for 30 minutes a day each day. Take stairs instead of elevators and park further away in parking lots. Wear a fitness gadget that tells you how many steps you achieve each day and always aim to beat the steps you took the day before.

Motivation is going to be key in your journey to better health. While working on your nutrition is the first step you need to take, becoming more active is going to allow your body to get stronger, become capable of withstanding new adventures, and quite frankly, will keep you from tiring out like you may do right now when long days or big events come your way.

Being “fit” doesn’t have to mean bench pressing your body weight at the gym (though that’s a great goal for anyone who’s interested). But what it does mean is that by being in better shape from where you are right now, your body will live longer, you will be healthier, your balance will get steadier, your flexibility will increase, your muscle mass will keep your bones and organs protected, you will burn fat, look better, and you will be able to live your life in a way in which you deserve to live it--without sitting back and watching others do the things you wished you could be doing.

Isn’t that in itself worth it?

The hardest part of any fitness routine is simply starting. The good news is that once you commit yourself, anything you do for roughly 21-30 days will become habit. Can you commit yourself to 30 days of moving more? Taking a few extra walks or doing a few sit-ups and squats before you shower each day? Yes, you can. I know you can. Because I had to do this once as well.

People who have met me within the last 10 or so years, don't really understand that I once needed a lot of motivation in my life. I was overweight, inactive, had no gym memberships, and I hated the thought of exercise. "Exercise is hard. I'm fat. I jiggle. People will laugh at me." My fitness journey has been a very long one, and it's crazy for me to sit back and think of how it started and how that led me to where I am right now. But the point is, I just had to get up off the couch and start. I committed myself over 10 years ago to stick with it, and now? There aren't many days in which I don't do at least something active--even if I can't get to a gym. At the minimum I will walk the dogs a mile or two. But I will move. If I can change my whole world (my career, my health, my life!) by committing to movement, you can too.

So let's start now, slow and steady, and see what you can do.

Let's assess your fitness and figure out how you should start.

Your Fitness Assessment

There are several ways to test your current ability, but these are very standard tests and should always be done in this order if possible:

The easiest way to assess yourself is to simply go to a doctor. You can go to your family doctor and get a physical (especially important if you haven't had one in a while), or you can get screened by a chiropractor or physical therapist who will check your movement patterns look for your weaknesses. Specialists such as these are great at providing you information on how to fix muscle imbalances, improve your range of motion, and ensure you have proper exercise form.

Test Yourself.

1. Assess your resting heart rate and blood pressure (if possible)

   a. Grab your true resting heart rate first thing in the morning when you wake up, BEFORE you get out of bed. Using your artery in your wrist, count the beats for one full minute. A normal heart rate is between 60-100 BPM and we'll use this number for a comparison against your cardiovascular test as well as a measurement for improvement in health.

b. If you are able to have your blood pressure taken by a professional, please do so. One in three Americans is borderline or has high blood pressure and you could be considered "at risk" for certain exercises. It's really important to know your blood pressure. Normal BP is typically 120/80.

2. Assess your body composition by using a skinfold caliper, waist-to-hip ratios, girth (circumference) measurements, or other readily available methods.

a. For a quick, at home assessment, the easiest way to do this, in my opinion, is with the waist-to-hip measurement. Studies show that the more fat that is stored in the waist area, the higher the person is at risk for diabetes, heart disease, and metabolic disorders.

b. The test is easy: divide the waist circumference (taken at the most narrow part of torso) by the hip circumference (taken at the maximum posterior protrusion of the buttocks). If the ratio is greater than or equal to 0.95 for men younger than 60 and 1.03 for men older than 60, the individual is considered obese. If the ratio is greater than or equal to 0.86 for a woman under the age 60 and 0.90 for women over 60, the individual is considered obese.

c. Keep a note of your measurements (and all your assessments) so you have something to compare to along your journey. One of the easiest ways to assess yourself is to take photos. Take some photos of yourself from the front, back, and sides. Continue to take progression photos each month. These are GREAT for being able to see the difference in your body--especially on days in which you are feeling a lack of motivation.

3. Assess your cardiorespiratory fitness by using the Rockport Walking Test.

a. The Rockport Walking Test is a great way to test your cardio health while getting a bit of decent exercise too! Simply warm up (lightly), and on a flat track or treadmill, walk one full mile at a quick pace. As soon as the mile is completed, immediately take your pulse using the artery in your wrist. Count for 10 seconds, then multiply that number by 6. Write this number down.

b. How does your heart health measure up? Use this online calculator to assess your health after your walk: http://walking.about.com/library/cal/ucrockport.htm.

4. Assess your muscular fitness with some push-ups! I know, it totally sounds like I'm making this up, but I promise I'm not. The easiest way to test your own muscular endurance is through a push-up test.

a. For men, a standard push-up is tested: on hands and toes--no knees. Perform as many standard push-ups as possible without rest at the top or bottom (bringing the chest about one fist-length away from the floor) and the test is over when no more push-ups can be performed with proper form.

b. For women, the same rules apply except all women must perform push-ups on her knees. (You can roll your eyes at this if you want. I did.)

c. Assess your muscular strength with the following chart:

	Age				
Rating	20-29	30-39	40-49	50-59	60+
MEN					
Excellent	>55	>45	>40	>35	>30
Good	45-54	35-44	30-39	25-34	20-29
Average	35-44	25-34	20-29	15-24	10-19
Fair	20-34	15-24	12-19	8-14	5-9
Poor	<19	<14	<11	<7	<4
WOMEN					
Excellent	>49	>40	>35	>30	>20
Good	34-48	25-39	20-34	15-29	5-19
Average	17-33	12-24	8-19	6-14	3-4
Fair	6-16	4-11	3-7	2-5	1-2
Poor	<5	<3	<2	<1	<0

And last, before you start any exercise routine, educate yourself on injury prevention! The last thing you ever want to do is get discouraged from exercising because you didn't know how to properly take care of yourself. Quitting exercise can quickly lead to depressive eating habits and the next thing you know, you're right back to square one. So read up!

By Strongfigure Ambassador & Coach, Kate Zanoni, LPTA

Whether you are a seasoned athlete or someone who is just starting out, it is important to practice injury prevention. Factors linked to workout-related injuries include overtraining, improper shoe support, muscle imbalances, inflexibility and insufficient recovery time.

The first step to preventing injury is to begin any new activity in moderation to avoid doing too much too soon. For instance, if you are a runner training for a marathon, you should slowly increase your mileage by a 10 percent incremental increase per week so your body can adapt to the increased mileage without the risk of developing overuse injuries. The same rule applies to any type of workout. It takes time to build your full potential regardless of whether you are a weekend warrior, routine gym rat or an exercise virgin.

Proper shoe support is vital to any workout regimen. It is essential to find a properly fitting shoe that meets your specific needs. Some people bear more weight on the inside of their feet (pronation), while others tend to roll ont o the outside of their feet (supination). Others have high arches that require more arch support. Regardless of your foot shape, gait pattern or your exercise of choice, finding the right support for your individual needs is crucial for avoiding easily preventable ankle, knee and hip injuries.

Muscle imbalances can be addressed by focusing on small muscle groups in addition to only training "mirror muscles" and large muscle groups. All too often, neglecting supporting muscle groups such as your individual scapular stabilizers, transverse abdominal muscles, internal and external hip rotators and intrinsic foot muscles (just to name a few) leads to injury in other areas of the body.

--Your scapular stabilizers are the muscles supporting your shoulder blades. This is an important muscle group to strengthen to avoid shoulder impingement and rotator cuff injuries.

--Your transverse abdominals run horizontally across your "core," creating 180 degrees of support for your spine. Training these muscles helps keep your spine healthy and decreases the stress on your lower back.

--Your internal and external hip rotators play a big role in the support and alignment of your pelvis and knee joints. Deficits in your hip strength can lead to injuries such as pelvic misalignment, back strains, and knee pain.

--Your intrinsic foot muscles aid in balance and play a role in how you stand, walk and run. When neglected, these weakened muscles will affect your proprioception, or your body's awareness of where you are in space. In turn, decreased proprioception affects your ability to balance properly while running, walking and even standing on uneven surfaces, increasing your risk for ankle injuries.

Inflexibility can be addressed with both dynamic stretches and static stretches. Dynamic stretches use momentum and should be performed as part of your warm-up to get your blood pumping while simultaneously preparing your muscles for activity.

Dynamic stretching, or stretching with movement, makes up the core of any warm-up because it activates the muscles you will use during your workout, improves your range of motion to help you feel more limber and improves your body awareness by challenging your balance and coordination. This will help maximize your overall performance whether you are hitting the pavement for a run, hitting the weights at the gym, hitting the mat for a yoga or Pilates class or hitting the field to play for your favorite sport.

Static stretching means gradually lengthening a muscle by holding it in an elongated position. Static stretches should be performed after activity as part of a cool-down routine to increase your overall tissue extensibility and decrease your likelihood for developing excessive post-workout muscle soreness known as delayed onset muscle soreness or simply, DOMS. Although considered a normal response to exercise, DOMS is muscle soreness you can experience beginning 12-24 hours after a workout and can last up to 72 hours. Excessive muscle soreness can lead to decreased performance. If left untreated, chronic tight muscles can lead to further damage to the affected muscle(s), causing injuries such as a muscle strain or even a tear. Static stretches should be held for a minimum of 20-30 seconds and repeated at least 3 times each for maximum tissue extensibility to prevent your muscles from re-tightening and rebounding like a rubber band.

Allowing sufficient recovery time is critical to avoiding injury. Build in at least one rest day per week to allow your muscles to recuperate. Pushing through pain and discomfort or overtraining will only lead you down the path to injury, forcing you to take an extended break from your favorite form of training while you restore your body back to health.

by Erik Walker

Our ancestors liked to walk. We were evolved to walk. And it is to this reason that we all should be walking a whole hell of a lot more than we do today. *Walking is the first and most important step to revamping your fitness.*

Did you know that anthropologists could tell if an ancient society were hunters and gatherers or farmers based on the density of their bones? Hunter-gatherer societies had strong dense bones because they were nomadic and spent much of their lives walking; whereas, farming societies had more brittle bones because they were more sedentary. Can you imagine what the future anthropologists will think of our bones?

We sit in our cars on the way to work, sit in front of a computer at work, sit again on our way home, where we sit down for dinner, and finally we sit in front of the TV as we unwind from our stressful day of sitting. Renowned physical therapist, Kelly Starrett, believes sitting is one of the least healthy positions we can put our body in--even going as far as saying that "sitting is the new smoking." Yet in 2017 America, we sit, sit, and sit some more.

The next time you sit in your car driving around a parking lot an extra 5 minutes looking for that super close parking spot so that you do not have to walk an extra 30 steps, think about what you are doing to your body.

Walking is undoubtedly better for you than sitting, and walking needs to be at the forefront of your journey to better health.

Walking is also the perfect accompaniment to a good muscle building resistance training program--which you'll learn about later. And since one of the keys to a healthier body is building muscle and maintaining a healthy weight, there really is no better combination.

A lot of your typical cardio exercise can actually slow the muscle building process, whereas walking can actually aid the muscle building process. Walking even stimulates blood flow which helps the muscles to recover from the resistance training.

More Reasons to Walk:

- A University of Michigan study found that outdoor walking can lower depression and decrease your stress levels. And reducing stress is one of the six essential keys to better health!

- Walking will also help you sleep better. A study published in the journal *Sleep* showed that women who added 3.5 hours of walking to their week slept better than women who did not.
- Walking is also the perfect starting point for your fitness journey. Walking is low impact so it has very little negative effect on the lower back, knees, and other problem areas associated with higher impact cardio.
- There have even been studies that have shown walking reduces fat at a higher rate than running and jogging!

And if that is not enough to convince you to start walking more, the American Heart Association says that walking 30 minutes a day can:

1. Reduce the risk of coronary heart disease
2. Improve blood pressure and blood sugar levels
3. Improve blood lipid profile
4. Maintain body weight and lower the risk of obesity
5. Enhance mental well being
6. Reduce the risk of osteoporosis
7. Reduce the risk of breast and colon cancer
8. Reduce the risk of non-insulin dependent (type 2) diabetes

"But I don't have time to walk!"

One of the big cons of walking is it is time consuming. This is certainly true and in our busy lives it often will become an excuse for not walking. But there are ways to make your walking more productive.

First, walking is an awesome relationship builder. Walking increases our mood and if you walk with loved ones, your brain begins to associate the feel-good hormones caused by the walk with the person you are walking with. So if you are trying to get someone to fall for you—take him or her for a walk.

Second, the average American watches 33 hours of television a week. Find a gym that has its treadmills in front of a TV. Some gyms have individual televisions for each treadmill. You can watch your favorite show while burning fat!

The benefits of walking certainly justify the 30-40 minutes of time it will take. Plus since your sleep will improve, you will be more rested and more productive throughout your day. So you may not even notice the extra 30 minutes taken from your busy life.

Still not convinced? Here are three more reasons:

1. Multiple studies have shown that walking improves your immune functioning. People who walk more get sick less.
2. According to the British Journal of Sports Medicine, walking improves your memory. Other studies have shown walking can improve other brain

functions as well, including lower your risks for dementia.

3. Finally, according to the National Walkers Health Study commissioned by the National Heart, Lung, and Blood Institute—walking has a direct association with a decrease in mortality—even amongst people who do other forms of exercise.

What is stopping you?

Walking is one of the easiest ways to improve your fitness, your health, and your life. We all know how to do it. So get started today. Below you will find two different 8 week treadmill walking workouts. The first program is a 4-day-a-week workout and is designed for a beginner who might be starting his or her new fitness journey with only walking.

The second program is designed for a beginner who is too busy for four days a week and/or is also incorporating one of our resistance training programs, which you will find later in this book.

Tips when beginning a treadmill walking workout:

- If possible, alternate the shoes you wear. This will save you from foot-related problems caused by walking.
- Massage your feet before and after by rolling a golf ball under your feet.

- Find a treadmill with an attached television or listen to your favorite podcast or audiobook while walking—the time will fly by and the distraction will make you forget you are working out.

Start Walking Now:

Here are two 8-week walking workout plans. The workouts in these plans are designed to keep your heart rate low and therefore in a greater fat burning zone.

	Day 1	Day 2	Day 3	Day 4
Week 1	20 minutes at 3.0 speed with no incline	20 minutes at 3.0 speed with no incline	20 minutes at 3.0 speed with no incline	20 minutes at 3.0 speed with no incline
Week 2	30 minutes at 3.0 speed with no incline	30 minutes at 3.0 speed with a 1.5% incline	30 minutes at 3.0 speed with no incline	30 minutes at 3.0 speed with a 1.5% incline
Week 3	30 minutes at 3.2 speed with no incline	30 minutes at 3.2 speed with 2% incline	30 minutes at 3.2 speed with no incline	30 minutes at 3.2 speed with 2% incline
Week 4	30 minutes at 3.3 speed with 1.5 % incline	35 minutes at 3.3 speed with 1.5 % incline	30 minutes at 3.3 speed with 2.5 % incline	35 minutes at 3.4 speed with 1.5 % incline
Week 5	40 minutes at 3.4 speed with 2% incline	40 minutes at 3.4 speed with 3% incline	40 minutes at 3.4 speed with 2% incline	40 minutes at 3.4 speed with 2% incline
Week 6	40 minutes at 3.5 speed with 2% incline	40 minutes at 3.5 speed with 3.5% incline	40 minutes at 3.5 speed with 2% incline	40 minutes at 3.5 speed with 2% incline
Week 7	40 minutes at 3.5 speed	40 minutes at 3.5 speed	40 minutes at 3.5 speed	40 minutes at 3.5 speed

	with 2% incline	with 4% incline	with 2% incline	with 2% incline
Week 8	40 minutes at 3.5 speed with 2% incline	40 minutes at 3.5 speed with 4.5% incline	40 minutes at 3.5 speed with 2% incline	40 minutes at 3.5 speed with 2% incline

Here is an 8 week three-day-a-week treadmill walking workout for the more time sensitive:

	Day 1	Day 2	Day 3
Week 1	20 minutes at 3.0 speed with no incline	20 minutes at 3.0 speed with no incline	20 minutes at 3.0 speed with no incline
Week 2	20 minutes at 3.3 speed with no incline	20 minutes at 3.3 speed with a 1.5% incline	20 minutes at 3.3 speed with no incline
Week 3	20 minutes at 3.5 speed with no incline	20 minutes at 3.5 speed with 2% incline	20 minutes at 3.5 speed with no incline
Week 4	20 minutes at 3.3 speed with 2.5 % incline	20 minutes at 3.3 speed with 2.5 % incline	20 minutes at 3.3 speed with 2.5 % incline
Week 5	20 minutes at 3.4 speed with 3% incline	20 minutes at 3.4 speed with 3.5% incline	20 minutes at 3.4 speed with 3% incline
Week 6	20 minutes at 3.5 speed with 4% incline	20 minutes at 3.5 speed with 4.5% incline	20 minutes at 3.5 speed with 4% incline
Week 7	20 minutes at 3.5 speed with 3% incline	20 minutes at 3.3 speed with 5% incline	20 minutes at 3.5 speed with 3.5% incline

Week 8	20 minutes at 3.5 speed with 4% incline	20 minutes at 3.5 speed with 4.5% incline	20 minutes at 3.5 speed with 4% incline

Walking Log Sheet

We have provided for you a printable Walking Log to help you track your daily walking at http://books.strongfigure.com/walking-log/.

The previous walking workout was designed to be completed on a treadmill and may be too difficult for some readers. If you find yourself in this position, here is a beginners walking workout that will get you up to walking an hour a workout in only 12 weeks:

Week	Sun	Mon	Tue	Wed	Thu	Fri	Sat
1	15 min	15 min	18 min	15 min	20 min	15 min	20 min
2	15 min	25 min	20 min	15 min	20 min	15 min	25 min
3	15 min	25 min	20 min	15 min	25 min	20 min	25 min
4	20 min	30 min	20 min	20 min	25 min	20 min	30 min
5	20 min	30 min	30 min	20 min	30 min	20 min	35 min
6	25 min	30 min	30 min	25 min	30 min	25 min	40 min
7	25 min	30 min	40 min	30 min	30 min	30 min	40 min
8	25 min	35 min	40 min	35 min	40 min	30 min	50 min
9	30 min	45 min	40 min	30 min	40 min	40 min	50 min
10	30 min	40 min	50 min	30 min	50 min	40 min	50 min
11	40 min	40 min	50 min	40 min	50 min	35 min	50 min
12	50 min	40 min	60 min	40 min	60 min	40 min	60 min

Walking With a Weight Vest

If you are looking for extra conditioning with your walking then you might want to try walking while wearing a weight vest. Wearing a weight vest while walking not only improves your conditioning but it will also increase the strength in your abdominal muscles, and your lower and upper back.

If this sounds good for you, I recommend purchasing a vest with adjustable weights. Most vests will allow you to add and remove weights. Anywhere from 10-30% of your bodyweight in pounds can be a good core workout.

My husband Erik and I typically wear a vest that is about 20-25% of our body weight and will walk between one and two miles with the vest every other day. On non-vest days we still walk! Walking every day is an essential part of your total body health.

There are many brands to choose from when choosing a vest, and we both have vests made by the brand MiR, and we have both been pleased.

Mobility

Since you're starting to become active, one key element to total body fitness is having a healthy movement pattern. Being flexible, learning how to stretch, and taking care of your joints are much more important than most people realize.

Whether you want to believe this or not, you need to take mobility as seriously as everything else you're doing to improve your health. If you do, you can avoid injury and you can seriously improve your body's flexibility, range of motion, balance, muscle recovery, and risk for tears, strains, sprains, and excessive soreness.

Stretching always seems to take a back seat to exercise. What's bad about this is that if you don't get in the habit of taking care of your joints, tendons, muscles, ligaments, etc., while you train; you may eventually hurt yourself. At the least, your muscles will tighten and knot up, and at the worst, you could tear a muscle, tendon, ligament, and may even need surgery.

Mobility is not an option. It's a MUST. It's part of training. It's part of life. Balance, flexibility, and mobility are a part of your journey and a part of being healthy for life. This is the key to successful exercise and training for life.

How Do You Become Mobile?

The first thing you need to do is stop sitting.

This is hard because most of us sit at work. If you can get up and stretch every 15 minutes throughout the day, you'll be ahead of the curve. Or if you can get up every 30 minutes and walk around for 5 minutes, you will be doing your body a tremendous favor. Since you've just introduced walking into your routine, by getting up and walking every 30 minutes or so, you're increasing your health AND improving your mobility. Famous mobility expert and doctor of physical therapy, Kelly Starrett, says that sitting is the smoking of our generation. Crazy, right?

The second thing you can do to become more mobile is to stretch! Whenever you can, stand up and stretch--just like you would when you get up in the morning. Walls and door frames are excellent for stretching! Grab hold of a door frame and turn away from it to stretch your chest. Put your toes up on the wall, bend your knee and stretch your calves and Achilles tendons. Prop your leg up on your chair to stretch your hamstrings, and then place your lower leg (think shoe to knee) across the top of your desk and lean forward to stretch your hips. In five minutes you can stretch your whole body in your office!

And if you're interested on how to overcome the pains of sitting, flag this article so that you can come back and access it anytime -- http://strongfigure.com/a-productive-pain-free-solution-for-sitting-all-day/

Take up yoga.

One simple way to increase your flexibility is by taking up yoga, and yoga is an excellent complement to walking and strength training--especially for beginners. Yoga will not only increase your flexibility and mobility but it'll help build some foundational strength for lifting weights. You don't have to necessarily take a 5-day-a-week yoga class, but learning a few poses that really help you hit the parts of your body that need a little extra stretching or strength can do wonders for both the body and mind.

Find a pose that helps you with your problem areas: shoulders, back, and hips, etc. Do these before and after you exercise in conjunction with a few wall stretches. If you have cable TV, you can probably find some yoga channels all set up and ready to teach you, or you could even buy a couple DVDs to have on hand. Your gym probably even offers yoga classes. Taking yoga even once a week will help improve your flexibility and keep your muscles and joints supple!

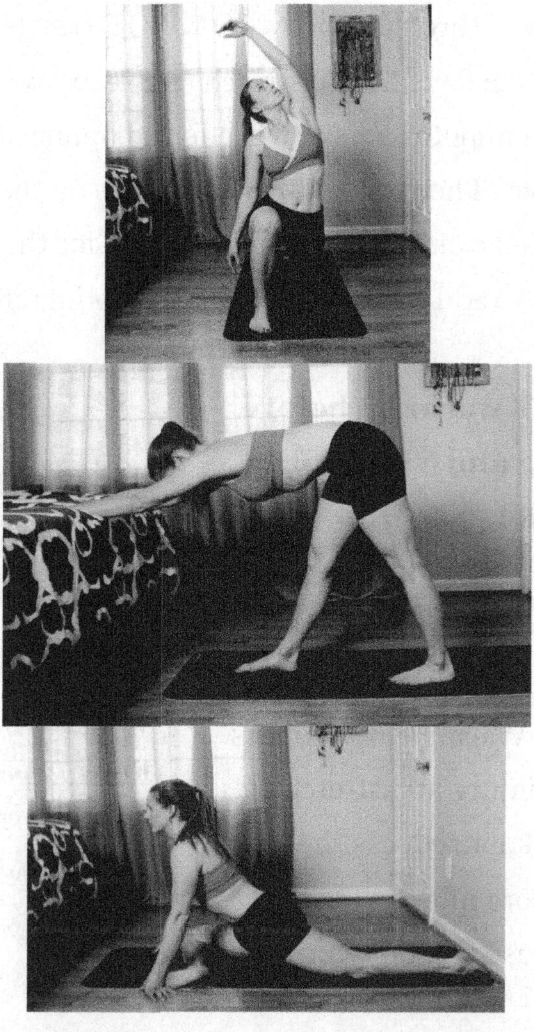

Strongfigure Ambassador, Reagan Theurer

Not into yoga? How about a Barre class? Barre fitness is simply a ballet-inspired class that mixes elements of Pilates, dance, yoga and functional training; and the moves are choreographed to motivating music.

One of my personal favorite ways to stretch and work on my mobility is through a daily ROMWOD (range of motion workout of the day). These stretch and relax workouts are typically 20 minutes long and are found online at romwod.com. They're PERFECT for those on the go and who just need a simple stretching routine for the end of a workout or to add to a daily routine for optimal flexibility.

You MUST warm up before exercising and STRETCH when done!

Try out a free two week membership to romwod.com by using this access code: **https://romwod.com/members/aff/go/strongfigure**.

Warming up and cooling down before any type of exercise is very important. Warming up reduces the risk of injury and stretching after a workout reduces the chance of sore muscles, as well as helps increase flexibility.

To warm up properly, you need to use "dynamic" movements--meaning moving stretches. I usually advise people to do whatever generates a light sweat--often times simulating what you're going to be doing for your workout, or doing a lower intensity workout--like a few air squats and push-ups--before starting the actual workout. Arm circles, leg swings--anything you can do to gradually start moving more and more and really get your body warm, loose, and open, will be just fine. Spend 5-15 minutes warming up (depending on your overall flexibility and mobility) warming up before starting any workout.

Having a tough time with flexibility?

The following seven poses are great for those who need a jump-start with increasing flexibility. These are also fantastic static stretches that you can use after your workout to help increase your flexibility.

1. Upper Chest and Back Opener: You can perform this stretch standing or sitting. Keeping your elbows bent, raise your arms to shoulder height and make hands into loose fists facing each other. Open your chest by drawing your elbows back as if you can get them to touch behind your back. When returning to the start position, continue the motion, as you wrap your hands around your opposite shoulders and stack your elbows on top of one another. To add on, you can get a nice stretch along upper back and the base of your neck by tucking your face into the space created by your elbows. Repeat the motion a second time, switching which elbow is on top. Do at least 2 to 3 sets.

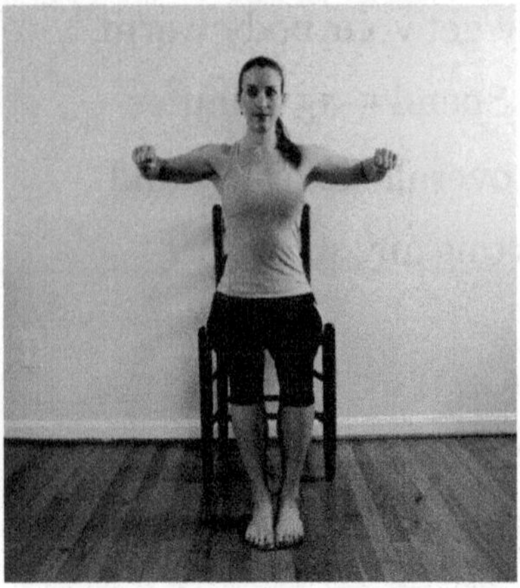

2. Standing Twist: Square your hips to the front of a chair, then place your right foot on the seat keeping your hips and thighs parallel to the floor. Then put your right hand on your hip and your left hand on your right knee and twist to the right. For a good counter twist, come back to the center and continue twisting to the left while placing your left hand on your hip and your right hand on your right knee. Repeat the twist/counter twist with your left foot on the chair. Make sure the twisting comes from the waist, and your hands should help hold you in the pose--not pull you into it.

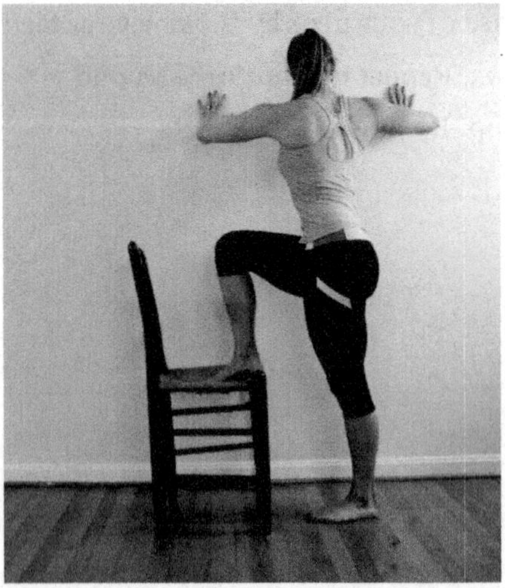

3. Half Dog: Stand a few feet in front of a wall and place your hands flat against the wall right at or a bit above waist height. Bend forward from the hips and then walk your feet back and continue to straighten out your arms. Don't arch your back and keep your tailbone neutral while your eyes gaze down. Start closer to the wall, or place your hands higher up if this 90-degree angle is too much. This pose is useful for easing you into the more traditional downward dog yoga pose. Hold for 2-3 deep breaths.

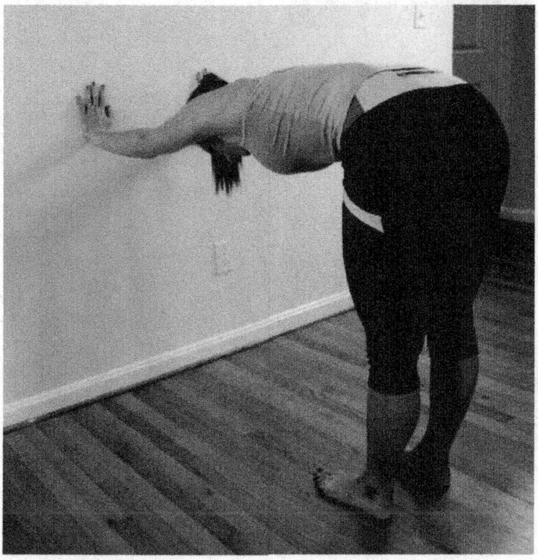

4. Chair-Assisted Half Dog: This is the same as the above half dog pose--it's just done with a chair instead of a wall. You can even do this stretch while holding onto a kitchen counter or your desk. Can you get more out of your body? If you feel good with your forward bends, try flipping the chair round and using the seat for balance. This will deepen the stretch and get you closer to touching your toes.

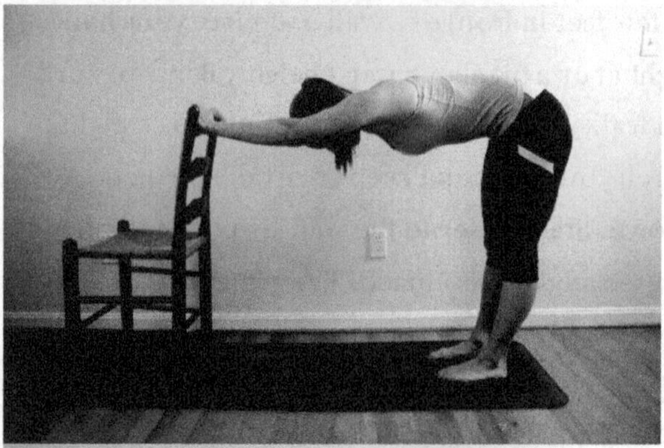

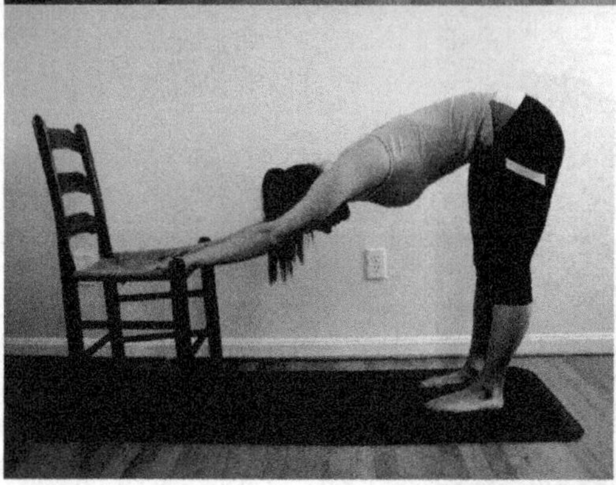

5. Seated Forward Bend Variation: This seated pose helps you gain flexibility in your lower body. Wrap a towel around your left foot and sit up straight. Bend your right knee and rest your right foot as far up left leg as right knee will allow. Bend forward from your hips. If your hamstring is too tight, hold the pose sitting upright. Hold for 2-3 breaths and repeat 2-3 times each leg. Not enough of a stretch? Try bending the elbows a bit to go a bit deeper into the bend. Repeat on the right leg.

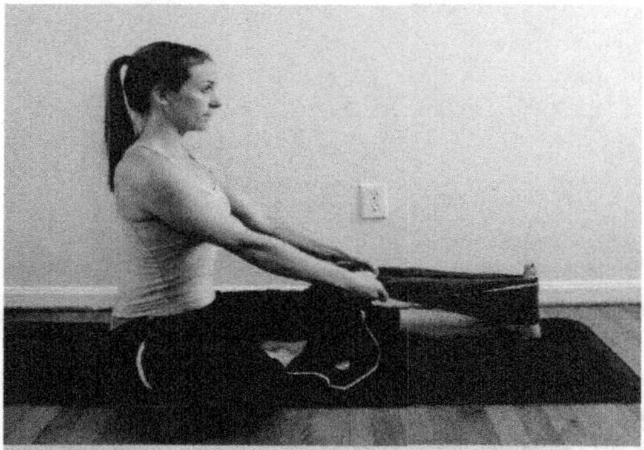

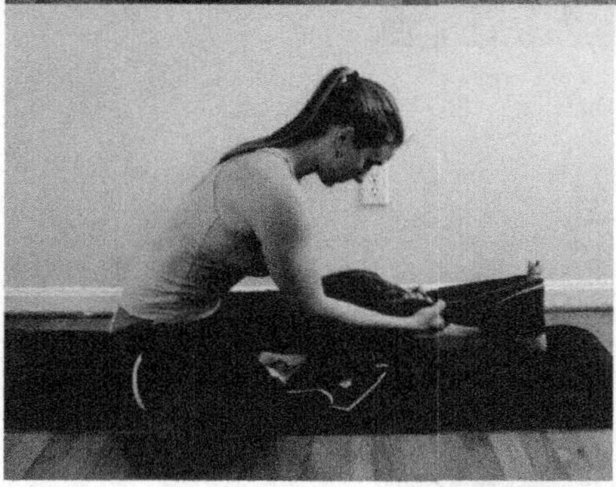

6. Reclining One Legged Stretch: This is one of the best hamstring stretches I know, and I help Erik with it all the time. Grab a chair, doorframe, (a person!) or the corner of a wall works well, too. Lie face-up on the floor, positioning body in a doorframe or up against a chair, so the right leg is on the ground through the doorway or on the floor, and left heel is positioned on the wall/chair. The closer your butt is to the wall/chair, the more intense the stretch--so if you're stiff, move your butt further away from the wall and position your left heel lower on the wall. Repeat on the right leg. Hold for 2-3 deep breaths and repeat 2-3 times each leg.

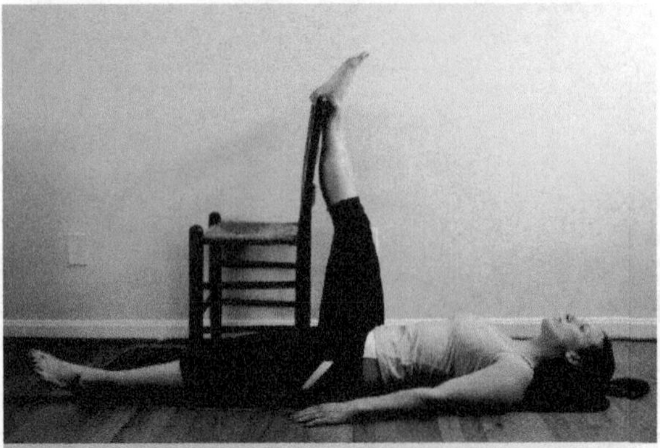

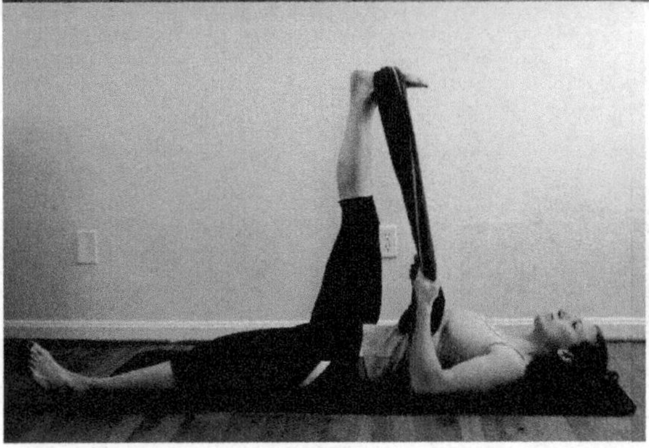

7. Easy Balance Sequence: Standing with a chair on left side, make sure your posture is in check and then with one or both hands resting on the chair back, raise your right foot in front of you a few inches off the ground and hold it there for three to five breaths. Bring the foot back into center, and then send it out to the side for three to five breaths. Bring your foot back into center, and then send it back behind you for three to five breaths. Repeat on the left leg. You can try this with one hand on the chair and bringing your foot to the side, or if you're feeling really balanced, try it without any chair at all!

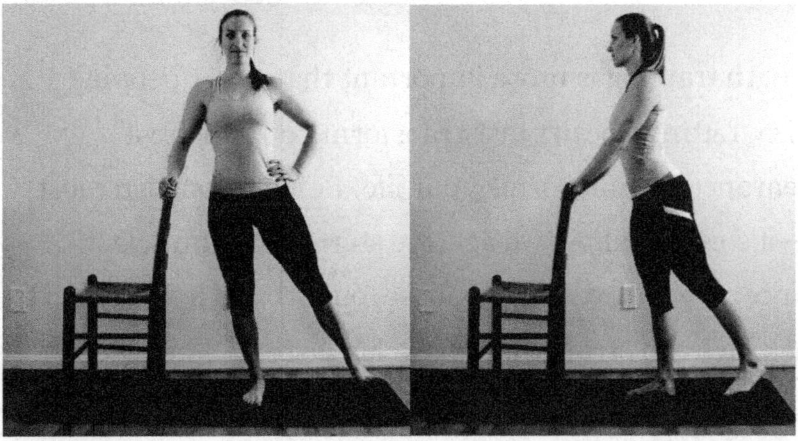

Extra stretching advice: Subscribe to ROMWOD.
I said it already, but my favorite way to stretch is by following the team at romwod.com. All you have to do is follow the video and practice holding stretches for 1-5 minutes per stretch. It may feel a bit advanced, however there are modifications for every level. It has personally done wonders for me--which is why I recommend it. Try out a free 14-day subscription here: https://romwod.com/members/aff/go/strongfigure.

Learning to Lift

You're walking. You're learning how to stretch and become mobile. But what if you want to do more than walk? What if you're in relatively good shape already? Or what happens when you want to add strength to your walking routine?

Strength training is more important than most people realize. Lifting doesn't just transform your physical appearance, it transforms your life. Being strong isn't just fun--it's essential. As we age, we start to lose muscle, balance, flexibility, and of course, our strength. If we don't attack life with strength, we lose life faster. Did you know that seniors, 65 and older, who suffer from a bad fall, are more likely to die within that same year? Do you know why seniors fall? Lack of muscle. Balance. Muscle protects your bones and organs. Muscle is more than just squats and deadlifts. Muscle burns fat and calories, but muscles also keep us safe, lean, and strong! Muscle is health!!

Lifting Programs

I have received AWESOME feedback from the three 12 week workout programs I designed for our Strong Figure Subscribers, so I have decided to include them here. There are three different levels:

- Beginners: 12 Week Beginners Workout
- Intermediate: 12 Week Intermediate Workout
- Advanced: 12 Week Advanced Workout

Choose the workout that best matches your current level of fitness. If you are reading this book on-line, each workout is complete with links to YouTube videos that further explain the exercises. If at any point you have trouble with an exercise, need a substitution, or do not understand, please send me a message at stephanie@stephaniewalker.net . I will try to answer your message as quickly as possible!

If you understand the importance of lifting weight, building muscle, and taking care of your body--but you're also scared of the weight room--here's a fantastic beginner's program to get you started. This is also perfect for the overweight novice lifter--nothing will start building muscle faster than some good ol' fashioned total body lifting.

The Novice Plan:

Monday	**Wednesday**	**Friday**
Leg Press 3x10	Romanian Deadlift 3x8	Goblet Squat 3x10
Bench Press 3x5	Strict Press 3x5	Push-Ups 3x Max Effort
Lat Pulldown 3x8-10 (overhand grip)	Lat Pulldown 3x8-10 (underhand grip)	Seated Rows 3x8-10
Plank Hold 3x Max Effort	Side Oblique Crunch 3x10-15 Each Side	Standing Lat Push Downs

		3x10-12

Instructional Help:

3x10 means that you will perform 3 sets of the exercise, 10 repetitions each. The weight should feel heavy enough that more than 10 reps would be a struggle to complete (with good form). You should feel like resting after your 10th rep--and do rest! Rest for a minimum of 30 seconds, up to 2 minutes. Then start set 2. Repeat for set 3.

The same applies for 3x8-10. Three sets of the exercise for 8-10 reps. Aim for 8 heavy reps. If you can get 10, great. If not, that's ok! The heavier you lift, the more you'll get out of your session and the faster you'll see results. This doesn't mean to go and injure yourself in the gym; just practice superb form with the heaviest weight that YOU can handle.

Expect to feel sore 1-2 days after training. If you train Monday--especially if new to training--you're likely going to feel sore on Tuesday. You may even feel worse on Wednesday. This is normal. Make SURE you stay hydrated, you stretch for at least 5-10 minutes before and especially after lifting, and you continue to stay mobile throughout the day. All these tips will help, including my favorite recovery method: a long, hot Epsom salt soak.

Sprinting and intervals are awesome.

But sprinting is not for everyone...yet. Many reading this book will need to start with walking and progress to lifting, and eventually add interval style bursts of high intensity exercises which can be accomplished through other forms of exercise, such as cycling and rowing. But when your body reaches the point that you can safely run and run hard—do it!

In a study on the impact of exercise intensity on body fat and metabolism, two groups of participants were put under two different exercise programs. One group did steady-state aerobic training for twenty weeks and one group did 15 weeks of sprint training (15 sprints for 30 seconds each), and the group that did the sprint training lost nine times more body fat.

Sprinting has shown to improve your body's ability to use and burn energy, thus improving your metabolism. Sprinting also increases musculature. Studies have shown that sprinting improves protein synthesis by as much as 230%.

Another study has shown that sprinting can also improve the body's ability to adapt to burning body fat for fuel. Most Americans have very high carbohydrate-based diets and the body loves carbohydrates for fuel. This is the reason many people have success in losing weight from following low-carbohydrate diets. By eating fewer carbohydrates, the body becomes more adapted to using body fat for fuel. However, this does not work unless you do the exercise to burn the body fat. In a study where subjects performed thirty second sprints on low carbohydrate diets, the fat burning increased by 75% and the fat burning continued two hours after the workout.

Do you need more incentive to sprint? In a 2011 study of overweight women, these women did short sprints on a stationary bike and showed a lower resting heart rate after only four weeks and a decreased risk of heart disease. And in a similar study, two groups, both with chronic inflammation, were given two different exercise regimens. The group that did sprint intervals showed a decrease in the inflammation that damages heart function compared to the group that did aerobic training.

One of the main reasons athletes jog is they believe it increases their endurance. But the body can actually increase endurance in a shorter amount of time though sprinting. This is because the body is amazing at adapting to sprint intervals and the body will begin to use energy more efficiently. A study showed that sprint intervals increased the amount of glycogen that can be stored in the muscles by as much as 20%.

Sprinting is also better at improving pulmonary lung function than steady-state cardio. In a study where one group performed five 60-second sprints with three minutes rest between each sprint for a total of twenty minutes, compared to another group that did steady-state cardio for the entire twenty minutes, the group that did the sprint intervals showed increased lung capacity and also had improved circulation compared to the steady-state cardio group.

A final reason people should sprint is because it increases brain functioning. In a vocabulary recollection study, a group which participated in intense sprint based workouts significantly outperformed a control group that did no exercise. Researchers believe intense exercise makes you smarter because it raises the hormones that stimulate the brain and increases neurotransmitters that are necessary for improved brain function. Sprinting decreases inflammation in the brain, improves the balance of hormones such as adrenaline that impact the brain, and stimulates dopamine which helps you to feel more energized.

Because sprinting is done for shorter periods of time, it causes less impact-related damage. And because sprinting requires an increased range of motion, it has less negative impact on your mobility. Actually, sprinting has been shown to increase mobility in long distance runners.

The benefits from a mix of sprinting and walking are outstanding. But transitioning from a walking program to a sprinting program may sound scary.

It's more than ok if you're not ready to hit the track for sprints. In fact, I'm not even sure it's a great idea to transition right from one to the other. So how do you make that switch? With interval exercise. Let's work on increasing your cardiovascular health and boosting even more muscle gains first. Once your heart is ready for sprints, then you can tackle as many of them as you desire!

High Intensity Interval Training (HIIT)

High intensity interval training works the same way that sprinting does. The only difference between "sprinting" and "HIIT" training is that you can use different exercises during your HIIT sessions. Instead of just sprinting, you could use kettlebell swings, dynamic lunges, burpees, wall ball exercises, etc., and this works for several reasons: People who train with intense intervals burn more fat while preserving lean muscle mass, improve cardiovascular/heart health, and increase their metabolism. The best part of interval training (as if the health benefits aren't enough) is that HIIT can be done almost anywhere at any time, and with most any exercise.

Most interval workouts take under 20 minutes to complete. HIIT increases your speed, decreases your fat, strengthens your core, gives you more power, allows for greater agility, and even builds muscle. And guess what else? It too, strengthens your heart. It's a no-brainer when it comes to choosing your conditioning training.

The workouts required for interval training are intense and much more challenging than one might expect. They're tough both physically and mentally. But the workouts are also much shorter (15-20 minutes long) and should only be completed 3-5 times a week–max. And of course you can start slow and build up–though intimidating, once you complete an interval workout, there's no greater feeling of accomplishment.

And the best news about interval training (besides the fact that it only takes 20 minutes?!) is that it burns twice as many calories as most other workouts. Once your twenty minutes are over, the body will actually continue to burn calories for up to 24-48 hours post-workout. When you endurance train, the calories stop when you do. Simple as that. But with interval training, the intense effort in which you put into your workout will cause your body to stay fired up for much longer. It's extremely similar to strength training.

Hello awesome metabolism!

Here are some other benefits of HIIT training:

- Interval training helps your heart rate peak, which will improve overall fitness, lung capacity, and muscle endurance.
- Interval training burns both carbs and body fat for fuel.
- Interval training burns calories longer than almost any other exercise.
- An interval workout is not only a quicker workout, but it works to burn fat quicker.
- In case you missed the last bullet, interval training helps you get lean, quickly!

It's a "no duh" answer on how to train. And quite frankly, it's how most everyone concerned with general fitness should train. Short, hard, and fast–that's it.

How to Start Your HIIT Training:

HIIT training is so versatile that there are many options on how to train in this style. Many people don't have an excessive amount of time to train every week, and some don't have more than thirty minutes a day. No problem. Find hills, run as fast as you can up the hill and walk or jog back down.

Another great option for intensifying your cardio would be by jump roping. A jump rope can be one of the cheapest pieces of cardio equipment that you can buy and it will work your total body from feet to shoulders. Try these two hoppin' combos guaranteed to get your heart rate bouncing:

The Fat Blaster:

- Jump for 30 seconds.
- Alternate leg jumps for 30 seconds. (Jump over the rope with one leg at a time.)
- Drop to the floor and perform 20 push-ups.
- Repeat the circuit two more times (3 total), rest for 60 seconds, then do it 3 more times. You'll end up completing the circuit 12 times with three rest periods.

The Heart Breaker

- 2 Minutes: Jump Rope

- 2 minutes: hold a plank (If you can't hold a plank on your toes for 2 minutes, use your knees until you can build up enough strength! Just keep your belly up!)
- Repeat this cycle for 90 seconds each exercise, 1 minute each exercise, and finally 30 seconds each exercise for a total of 10 minutes.

If jump-roping isn't your thing, one of my favorite ways to strength train AND boost my cardio performance is the **Tabata Method**. A tabata can be done with ANY exercise, and it only takes 4 minutes per exercise. Four! All you have to do is pick as many exercises as you'd like to do (four exercises is standard for a 16 minute workout).

Let's say you choose kettlebell swings, burpees, bodyweight squats, and pushups. Start with the swings, and swing for 20 seconds and rest for 10. Repeat (8 times total) for a total of four minutes all together. Move straight into the next exercise. It sounds much easier than it is. **Tabatas ROCK.** And because you can choose whatever exercises you do with them, your workout will never get boring. Try squat jumps, lunges, triceps dips, pull-ups, burpees–it doesn't matter. You'll advance your cardio and improve your strength and endurance. Isn't that what matters?

HIIT Workouts that will boost metabolism shrink waistlines:

Here are four pyramid-style interval workouts designed to leave you fitter, faster, and well, totally flustered when done.

Workout One. Complete:

- 100 jumps with a jump rope
- 75 body weight squats
- 50 push-ups
- 25 burpees

Workout Two. Complete:

- 10 burpees
- 10 sit ups
- 9 burpees
- 9 sit-ups
- 8 burpees
- 8 sit ups
- 7 burpees
- 7 sit-ups....all the way down to 1 and 1

Workout 3. Complete:

- 10 push-ups
- 10 bodyweight squats
- 100 meter sprint
- 9 push-ups
- 9 squats
- 100 meter sprint.....all the way down to 1, 1, and the last 100 meter sprint

Workout 4. Complete:

- 21 Body weight squats and push-ups
- 15 squats and push-ups
- 9 squats and push-ups

Here are five "3-Rounds for Time" workouts equally designed to kick your booty:

Workout 1. 3 Rounds:

- 20 jumping jacks
- 20 burpees
- 20 bodyweight squats

Workout 2. 3 Rounds:

- Run 400 meters
- 50 bodyweight squats

Workout 3. 3 Rounds:

- 30 push-ups
- 30 second wall-sit hold
- 30 alternating lunges (option is to hold weight if possible)

Workout 4. 3 Rounds:

- Run 200 meters
- 25 push-ups
- 25 squats

Workout 5. 3 Rounds:

- 20 squats
- 20 burpees
- 20 push-ups

- 60 second plank

But these seem harder than what I'm ready for!

These workouts probably look pretty tough. That's ok--they are. I want to challenge as many people as I can. That doesn't mean you have to do every workout as it's written. Cut the reps in half or substitute a different movement. If you're not ready to sprint but you're able to do the rest of the workout, substitute walking for the sprints. You do what YOU have to do in order to boost your fitness. Just keep moving. As long as you're moving, you're improving your health.

Sprint Workouts:

Once you've conquered intense interval cardio, you're ready to start sprinting. This can be where you'll excel in REVAMPing your fitness!

Sprint with Caution

Like I mentioned earlier, sprinting can be hard on the body if you are a beginner. I would start implementing the theories of sprinting on a stationary bike or stationary rower, first.

Here are some tips to help sprint safely:

- Warm up to a light sweat and then stretch the leg muscles and torso muscles using a combination of static and dynamic stretching.
- Always do at least three short 50%-75% (effort) warm-up runs before sprinting.
- Sprinting on a hill or incline will prevent over striding and will decrease the risk of hamstring injuries.
- Sprint on soft surfaces such as grass as you build up the muscles to be able to handle sprints.
- Remember that you should never sprint at full speed unless you are completely warm and stretched. It is important to not over stride, keep your feet in a singular line, and build your momentum slowly to avoid muscle tearing.

Here's one of my favorite sprint workouts that I have used probably hundreds of times in my own training. It takes 15 minutes and you can do this on a track or a treadmill.

- Jog 30 seconds, sprint 20 seconds
- Jog 1 minute, sprint 30 seconds
- Jog one and half minutes, sprint 40 seconds
- Jog 2 minutes, sprint 50 seconds
- Jog 2 and a half minutes, sprint 1 minute
- Jog 3 minutes sprint 1 minute and 10 seconds

Total: 15 minutes. You should feel out of breath when done. It's complete hell but it also works. Besides, wouldn't you rather do cardio for 15 minutes instead of an hour?

400s Rock

As with sprinting, 400s can be hard on the body, especially if you are in poor shape. If you are in an average beginner shape, you can get tremendous benefits from 400 meter runs; however, you must make sure to use caution and warm up properly! If you're not in average shape already, you can reach this level and achieve a similar workout on a stationary bike or rower just by biking or rowing as fast as you can for sets of 20 second sprints (with one minute rest period) and repeat.

Start with 20 second intervals and build up to 30 seconds, then 45 seconds, and all the way up to a minute plus. When you can start doing minute long sprints on the rower or bike, you are ready for the track!

A 400 is one lap on a standard track. 400s are a virtual sprint. Yes, you are sprinting for an entire lap. This may feel terrible, but these sprints are probably one of the most amazing exercises you can do for both your overall health and your physical appearance.

To do 400s correctly you do need to be timing yourself. 400s are to be run FAST so that you will want to challenge yourself and try to set new personal records. For example, let's suppose you are a fairly athletic female and the first time you try out a 400 workout you are able to run it in 90 seconds. Set 70-75 seconds as your personal goal. Men on average will be about 10-15 seconds faster than women. So the same male athlete might go out and run a 75 second 400, and his goal would be to finish a 400 in 60 seconds.

Before you start thinking this is way too fast, just remember this is just a matter of training for it and doing it. The timer and goal setting will force you to be running your 400s at the speed they need to be run.

"I discovered the high fat burning potency of 400m sprints without really looking for it. I use a lot of 400m running with my hockey players, mostly because it develops the energy system they require most during a game. However, I quickly noticed how lean they were getting shortly after starting 400m runs. Furthermore, they were getting leaner and stronger! I then experimented with 400m for fat-loss purposes and found time after time how efficacious it truly was. To this day I still believe that few things can match up with 400m runs for fat loss." -- Christian Thibaudeau

Get Your Miles Workouts through Sprinting and Walking and HIIT Work!

Workout A:

- 100 meter sprint followed by 300 meter walk
- Repeat 16 times. (This is a four mile workout and it can be shortened to lower repetitions if your conditioning is not ready for 16 100-meter sprints)

Workout B:

- Eight 200 meter sprints followed by 200 meter walks -- depending on your conditioning, make sure after each walk, your heart rate is at near resting rate before beginning your next sprint. If you cannot sprint for 200 meters then only do workout A.

Workout C: (this one is only for the well-conditioned)

- Four 400 meter sprints--walk until fully recovered. It is very hard to sprint for 400 meters so if you are not fully sprinting then stick with workout A or B

14 Sprint & Conditioning Workouts

Some of these workouts are pretty advanced so start slow and modify as you need. If you're just getting started, just do what you can. Sprint to you may mean something different to the more conditioned athlete. That's ok! You're here to improve your fitness and if you didn't have any areas for improvement, you'd have no goals to set and nothing to work towards. You just start where you need to and you'll build up in no time.

4 Rounds for time:

- 400 meter sprint (.25 on t-mill)
- 1 minute plank

4 Rounds for time:

- 400 meter sprint
- 2 minute rest

9 Rounds for time:

- 60 second jog
- 30 second sprint

10 Rounds for time:

- .10 treadmill sprint (100 meters)
- Rest the same amount of time it took to sprint 100 meters

Complete the following for time:

- .20 treadmill (or 200m) sprint, 4 minute rest
- .20 sprint, 3 minute rest
- .20 sprint, 2 minute rest
- .20 sprint 1 minute rest
- .20 sprint, done

3-5 Rounds for time:

- 10 kettlebell swings
- 10 burpees

5 Rounds for time:

- .20 sprint
- 10 burpees

For 15 minutes:

- sprint for 15 seconds
- rest for 45 seconds

5 Rounds for time: 3-5 Rounds

- .15 sprint
- 15 kettlebell Swings
- 1 farmer carry lap around track=heavy!
- 10 push-ups
- 1 sprint around track

For 12 Minutes:

- sprint for 30 seconds
- rest for 30 seconds

3 Rounds:

- 25 kettlebell swings
- 25 burpees

For 20 Minutes:

- 30 seconds sprint
- 60 seconds rest

For 8 Minutes:

- sprint for 20 seconds
- rest for 10 seconds

For 20 Minutes:

- sprint for 1 min (maximum effort)
- rest for 2 minutes

To help you keep track of these workouts, you can find a printable workout log here:

http://books.strongfigure.com/strong-figure-conditioning-workout-log/

If you are at a more advanced level, then you might want to look into adding some of the kettlebell workouts from 100 Hours of Kettlebells to your weekly routine. Many of these workouts are very difficult and very intense so these should be reserved for the more conditioned athlete. If you do decide to purchase 100 Hours of Kettlebells use the promo code: subscriber100kb (25% off).

How to Monitor Your Heart:

One way to ensure that you aren't overworking yourself–even for the most advanced athletes–is to monitor your heart rate. If you subtract your age from 220, the number you get is the number that your heart rate should never exceed. When interval training, your goal will be to reach this number during your periods of "work" and then rest only long enough to drop the number back closer to where you started. Sooner or later, the time it takes to lower your heart rate back to normal will get shorter and shorter–showing you the effective results of interval training on the body. Your heart will get stronger and your recovery time will decrease.

How to find out your heart rate? When working out, stop and for 10 seconds, count the number of times you can feel your pulse beating in your wrist. Multiply this number by 6 and that should give you your current heart rate. Remember that it should never get over your calculated number that you figured out above.

To Recap...

The good thing about sprinting and interval training is that they are both extremely flexible and can be done with almost any exercise. The goal is to get the heart rate elevated–ensuring max effort on your part–and then bringing it back down to recover. This constant work/rest fluctuation is what makes the body stronger and more efficient. If you've never tried interval training before, or especially if you're new to working out at all, please start slow!

The last thing you want to do is scare yourself away from what can be one of the best ways to exercise. It sometimes happens–a person works SO hard on his or her first HIIT session that he decides it was "too" hard and never does it again. It's totally ok to start slow. Everyone must learn to doggie paddle before jumping off the high dive.

Other Ways to Increase Your Activity: AKA--DO RAD SH*T!

In 2015, my husband Erik developed a campaign for our fitness site, Strongfigure. He called it, "Do Rad Sh*t." Simply, he wanted to show that world that being "Fit" doesn't have to mean deadlifting 300 pounds, it means enjoying life the way you want to. It means not having to sit on the sideline while the rest of your family or friends go on vacation and they want to walk the beach but you can't. It means doing what you want when you want to do it, all because you CAN. You can go wake-boarding or stand-up paddle boarding because you're healthy and fit enough. You can DO RAD SH*T.

Why should this matter?

I once worked with a woman who came to me and said, "I just want to be able to keep up with my family when we go on vacation." She was an obese lady in her 40s and I could tell how sad she was. She said that if her family went shopping, she had to rent an electric cart in order to keep up with them. On vacation, they would have to stop and let her sit if they tried to go for a walk anywhere. Many times, she said, they just left her behind. She couldn't walk with her family.

I'm sad writing this. No one should have to live this way! Eating wholesome foods and accomplishing 60 minutes of activity each day does NOT have to be hard!

You don't have to buy a gym membership in order to become healthier. You don't have to do even half of the exercises I listed previously. I wholeheartedly believe that

- walking
- basic strengthening exercises (including yoga and bodyweight movements like squats, sit-ups, push-ups, etc.), and
- mobility (again yoga or simple stretching)

are enough to keep anyone in decent shape. Adding the extra weights and interval training just increases overall effort and quickens the effects of fat loss, heart health, and all the great benefits that come with added muscle and exercise.

But just getting up and out and doing something fun--by yourself or with your family--can improve your health more than you know! Do any of these sound fun to you?

- Hiking
- Camping
- Swimming
- Going to the park with your kids
- Playing disc golf
- Roller skating
- Canoeing
- Gardening
- Skiing
- Adult Gymnastics or Adult Dance
- Walking your dog(s)

You could volunteer services at an animal shelter and take dogs out to play, clean kennels. You could go out and pick up trash along the road on which you live. How can you improve your community or the lives of others while getting fitter along the way?

Google the city in which you live and see what pops up as attractions or adventures. See if you have a local Parks and

Recreation that may offer classes and activities at reduced rates. My rec center offers fitness classes, dance, gymnastics, yoga, pickleball, volleyball and basketball. It even has a senior wellness program. And some of these are free to participate in and the rest are really inexpensive. So go out there and check out what your community has to offer. You never know what you may end up finding!

Before moving on, I want you to answer these questions:

1. What are you going to do so that you can start moving more each day?

2. How/when are you going to accomplish this goal?

"I will sleep when I'm dead."

"Sleep is for the weak."

With mantras like this, is it any wonder why 100 million Americans are chronically sleep deprived? Sleep deprivation is dangerous for your body, dangerous for your mind, and dangerous for society. Lack of sleep can lead to weight gain, hypertension, anxiety, and depression.

Sleep is Important

- When we sleep our brains flush out harmful neurotoxins.
- During sleep we consolidate memories and reinforce learning.
- During sleep we repair our bodies.
- When we sleep we fight off infection and disease.
- And during sleep we replenish hormones and neurotransmitters.

Generally, we put our body in a physiological state to be ready for the next day. If we do not sleep we are not in a physiological position to be successful in our daily tasks.

A study done by the American Academy of Sleep Medicine found that morning people and people who got at least 7 hours of sleep a night also ate healthier than those who slept in and those who slept less.

Late nighters crave sugar and fatty foods that give them energy. But those early morning folks have plenty of energy and therefore do not have the need for those bad-for-you foods.

And according to fittnessmagazine.com, morning people are happier, suffer from less stress, are more productive at work, are more alert and reliable, and they lose more weight. Most of these accomplishments occur because those who rise early simply get things done. They exercise earlier and set the tone for the day. They are motivated and therefore make better food decisions.

Most morning people plan their day and make lists and write down daily and weekly goals. And according to a study done by University of Toronto researchers, morning people actually tackle their hardest tasks first thing–when people (morning or not) are at their peak efficiency. Morning people just have their sh*t together, okay?

Sleep's Impact on the Body and Athletic Performance

- Sleep deprivation slows glucose metabolism by as much as 40%. No one wants a slow metabolism.
- Sleep deprivation increases cortisol, a stress hormone which directly affects body fat storage and weight gain. Individuals with elevated cortisol levels are at a greater risk for weight gain and obesity.
- Lack of sleep also leads to insulin resistance, a condition in which your cells do not use insulin properly. There is a direct connection between type 2 diabetes and insulin resistance.
- Sleep deprivation causes a decrease in growth hormone, which is necessary in tissue repair. Athletes with chronic soreness and inflammation can often trace this to sleep related issues.
- Poor sleep leads to decreased glycogen synthesis. Glycogen is the body's energy source for intense exercise, such as sprinting and weightlifting. Glycogen helps break down fat into energy the body can use. A decrease in glycogen synthesis also adds more work and stress on the kidneys. When the body does not properly synthesize glycogen, it will begin using proteins for energy which are harder for the kidneys to process. Many of us may have adequate glycogen storage but our bodies do not synthesize it properly—one reason for this may be sleep deprivation.
- Lack of sleep also increases cravings for sugar and high caloric foods. In one study, subjects would sleep for 8 hours a night and then have their next day food choices recorded. Then they slept for four hours and had their next day food choices recorded. After the four hour sleep night, participants ate more calories and showed preferences for high calorie junk foods.

- A University of Colorado study found that just losing a few hours of sleep in consecutive nights led to a weight gain average of two pounds.
- One study showed sleep restricting young, healthy, college-age students for just four days resulted in blood glucose and insulin levels consistent with those suffering from obesity and diabetes.
- Both adults and children are more likely to be overweight the less they sleep.
- Sleep deprivation increases our risk for accidental injury and accidental death.
- Chronic sleep deprivation increases our risk for almost every disease -- cancer, heart disease, strokes, obesity, and diabetes.

Sleep's Impact on the Brain and Cognitive Function

- Studies show sleep deprivation hinders working memory.
- Lack of sleep also affects your ability to pay attention.
- Sleep deprivation impairs visuomotor performance, an important aspect of cognition.
- Sleep deprivation impairs the brain's reasoning ability.
- Sleep deprivation also negatively affects both long term and short term memory.
- Sleep deprivation has a tremendously negative effect on all cognitive function. In addition to the aforementioned examples, lack of sleep increases perseveration errors (repeating words or phrases), rigid thinking, and poor sleep can increase difficulty in using new information necessary for decision making and solving complex tasks.

- Lack of sleep can cause depression and even increases the risk for suicide.

Sleep's Impact on Society

The fact that sleep wrecks our health, causes depression, and hurts our relationships proves that lack of sleep has a negative effect on society. But when we look at how sleep affects our daily performance, things get even scarier. 100 million Americans get poor sleep. The average American sleeps 6.5 hours a night, which is 20% less than we slept just 30 years ago.

Why is this such a major concern?

Research shows that being awake for 18 hours in a day has the same effect as a blood alcohol content (BAC) of .05 -- the legal limit of intoxication in most of Western Europe and Australia. In one study, participants who were awake for 21 hours performed worse on simple cognitive and motor tasks than participants who had a BAC of .08. Being awake for 24 consecutive hours has the same performance effect of a BAC of .1.

One third of Americans are essentially living out their lives with the same performance abilities of people who are intoxicated. Our doctors, policemen, teachers... all doing their daily duties and tasks at the equivalence of someone who is drunk. The business and financial world estimates $200 billion annually in lost production due to poor sleep.

Do You Suffer From Poor Sleep?

Sleeping more requires a tremendous commitment. You have to change your entire value system and you have to challenge the current social norms that are forcing so many Americans into chronic sleep deprivation. Most who suffer from poor sleep think they are fine. In fact, in most of the sleep restriction studies, the participants reported feeling fine. Sleep is a silent killer.

But how do you know if you are getting enough sleep?

Dr. Deborah Gordon uses this checklist to assess whether her patients are getting adequate sleep:

1. Are you sleeping 8-9 hours a night?
2. Are at least 4-5 hours deep sleep?
3. Do you remember some of your dreams?
4. Do you wake feeling refreshed?

If you answered, "Yes" then you are one of the lucky ones who are getting enough sleep. But for many, sleep is a luxury. Sleep is something many wish that they had but just don't know how to get it, or worse, isn't believed to be the priority it is.

But what if you are part of the population who biologically suffers from poor sleep? Meaning you *try* to get good, adequate, well-rested, deep sleep; however, biologically you and maybe even some people in your family just struggle with sleep--no matter what?

Nearly nine million U.S. adults depend on prescription sleeping pills to get sleep. But sleeping pills do not work. Yes you may sleep, but the purpose of sleep is to allow the body to be in a physiological state in order to thrive the next day. Sleeping pills restrict these physiological benefits. Essentially, we might as well not sleep.

So what can be done?

Supplements

In our experience, most supplements do not work for sleep acquisition or they only work for a short period of time. The best success Erik (who has had poor sleep issues his whole life) ever had with a supplement for sleep was a night time protein drink made by Progenex called **"Cocoon."** Cocoon contains L-tryptophan, (yes the stuff in turkey that makes you sleepy on Thanksgiving) and it worked great for a few months, but then he started having diminishing returns. Essentially, it stopped producing great nights of sleep. We have talked with a few others who had similar results. They loved it but then Cocoon eventually stopped working.

He has also tried supplementing with **melatonin** (the sleep hormone), and he had decent success. However, there is a growing amount of evidence showing that if you take melatonin, your body will stop naturally producing it. The scientific community seems to be in debate over this, but to me, it's not worth the risk that your body might stop producing a necessary hormone for sleep.

Tart cherry is a really popular option and I have heard people rave about its sleep benefits. Tart cherry purportedly increases your natural melatonin production. Sadly, Erik and I have wasted quite a lot of money in health stores buying various forms of tart cherry with very little success.

ZMA is a supplement we would recommend with caution to someone struggling with sleep. ZMA (or zinc monomethionine and aspartate and magnesium aspartate) is a supplement with considerable research showing its effectiveness. Unfortunately, Erik's overly regular digestive system cannot handle ZMA. Magnesium can have a laxative effect on the intestines and many report such effects from ZMA usage.

There are some doctors who will suggest avoiding magnesium aspartate because it breaks down into aspartic acid, which can be toxic. But I have also heard the magnesium aspartate binding to the other ingredients in ZMA minimizes this risk.

I have known athletes who have taken ZMA for years and swear by it. There is also considerable empirical evidence to its effectiveness, but remember it can cause diarrhea in some users and there are some doctors who will tell you to avoid magnesium aspartate.

The absolute number one supplement that anyone suffering from sleep-related problems should take is **vitamin D**. Vitamin D, taken in the morning, can greatly improve the body's physiological ability to produce quality sleep. According to the federal government's National Health and Nutrition Examination Survey, as many as 75% of all Americans are deficient in vitamin D. Vitamin D has been shown to help with natural melatonin production and vitamin D is necessary in maintaining optimal hormone levels.

There are other supplements out there that promise sleep (such as glycine, magnesium, and bedtime teas) but these five are the only ones that I have come across that have anecdotal and empirical evidence supporting their effectiveness. However, it should be noted that Erik does not use any supplements, other than vitamin D, to aid him in his sleeping issues. Also noted--we are not registered dieticians and cannot prescribe supplements to anyone. We can, however, bring you research and help educate you with information you need to make decisions on your own. When it comes to sleep and supplements, we know how different each person and each body is. Take the time to experiment on your own and find something that works best for YOU.

Erik's solution, and hopefully yours, will be to improve your SLEEP HYGIENE.

Erik's Sleep Hygiene

If you are serious about getting good quality sleep, here are nine sleep hygiene strategies:

1. **Schedule.** In my experience, the number one most effective sleep tool is sticking to a schedule. This will be difficult in the beginning and it may mean sacrificing a few hours of sleep at first. But schedule a wake time and never vary from that time by more than an hour. So if you set 6:30 am as your wake time then you should never get up earlier than 5:30 am and never get up later than 7:30 am. Some experts recommend never varying by more than 30 minutes. I will be honest; it is hard to do this on weekends. I have to get up at 6 am on weekdays. When my alarm rings at 7 am on a Saturday, it is difficult to convince myself that getting up right now will help my sleep.

2. **Darkness and light.** Before bed the body cannot produce sufficient melatonin in the light.

When it is time to sleep, you need darkness. Avoid lights, especially blue light at least one hour before it is time to sleep. Use bright light to wake yourself. In fact, exposure to sunlight early in the day will increase your vitamin D levels and actually aid in your sleep. Vitamin D deficiency is very common and I would highly recommend that you supplement with vitamin D in the morning. There is evidence that sunlight exposure early in the day also increases melatonin production.

3. Silence. Many have success with white noise, music, or sleep machines. If you do rely on such devices, have them set on a timer to go off. Most sleep experts suggest that quiet sleep produces more REM and overall better sleep.

4. Avoid Blue Light. Cell phones, tablets, computer screens, and televisions all emit a blue light that blocks the brain's production of melatonin. Many experts suggest avoiding all such screens for three hours before bed. In doing research for this chapter, I have heard many anecdotal reports stating that wearing blue blocker glasses at night has greatly improved sleep for many individuals. I ordered a pair for myself and they do in fact work; however, they may pose as more of an inconvenience for many people. I also recently learned that just by having your electronics turned on in your bedroom can hinder your sleep. If you sleep next to your phone at night, turn your phone on airplane mode and turn everything else off!

5. Cooler temperatures. The body sleeps better in cool temperatures. Do not work out right before bed or take hot baths as both of these activities will raise your core body temperature.

6. Caffeine. Caffeine affects everyone differently, but if you have any issues with sleep, you should avoid all caffeine 8 hours before bed. You CAN, however, use caffeine in the morning to help wake yourself up! If you're struggling to form a morning routine, caffeine doesn't deserve the bad rep it sometimes gets. Drink your cup of coffee, (or tea, and preferably without the sugar) and have a tall glass of water with it. For non-morning people, this can be a huge help.

7. Alcohol. Alcohol decreases quality sleep and too much alcohol may block all REM sleep. Excessive alcohol has a similar effect as sleeping pills. This is not quality sleep and the body and brain will not get the physiological effects of deep sleep from the type of sleep induced from alcohol.

8. Exercise. Most studies show that exercise does indeed improve sleep. Just remember to not exercise too vigorously right before bed. The rare exception to exercise helping with sleep is if you have an adrenal/cortisol problem. If you suspect you may have such a problem you should consult a doctor.

9. Blood sugar balance. Too much insulin can drive your blood sugar levels to drop at night, which will lead to restless sleep. To avoid this, eat healthy blood sugar balancing foods such as grass-fed beef, shellfish, fish, vegetables, and plenty of quality fat, such as fat from butter, avocado, coconut oil, animal fat, and fish oil. Avoid too many grains, sugar, and only eat small amounts of fruits at night, as these foods can upset your blood sugar balance.

There are some other potential health concerns that could be affecting your sleep. Thyroid issues, low testosterone in men, and suboptimal levels of estrogen in women can also lead to poor sleep. Please consult a physician if you think you may suffer from any of these problems.

Bonus Sleep Tips:

- **Make bone broth.** Many experts recommend consuming bone broth for better sleep. Bone broth is high in glycine, which is an amino acid known to help with deep sleep. Bone broth is easy to make and is one of the most nutritious foods you can consume for overall body health.

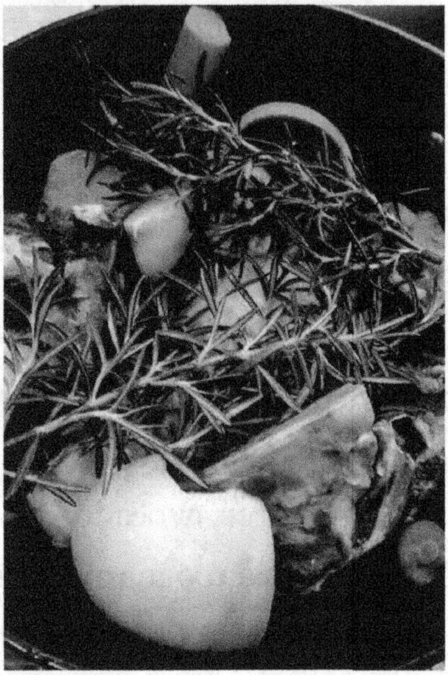

Easy Beef Bone Broth Recipe:

- 5-8 lbs of beef bones
- Lots of veggies--your choice! Most people choose carrots, onion, and celery.
- Enough water to cover the bones
- Sea salt, garlic, and any other herbs you want to use to flavor your broth
- 2 TBS Apple Cider or Balsamic Vinegar to ensure that you pull the minerals out of the bones.
- 1-2 bay leaves
- Rinse and dry the bones, then roast for about an hour at 400 degrees until the bones are brown. Keep the fat that drains off the bones!

- Add all your ingredients to stock pot or crockpot--the bones, fat, veggies, spices, everything but vinegar and bay leaves--and cover with water.
- Bring the water to a boil and then add vinegar and a bay leaf or two.
- Turn heat to a simmer and let the pot cook for 8-12 hours if on the stove, 12-24 if in a crockpot.
- When done, you'll have to filter out the stock and store into containers. Some people like to use mason jars--I like to use Ziploc bags so I can write on the bags and store them in the freezer.

You can do the same thing with chicken bones! And if you can find them, use chicken feet and necks for added nutrients.

- **Yoga for sleep.** I have actually tried this tip and I think it does work in that it lowers your stress at night and reduces the running-mind phenomenon that many blame for their poor sleep.

Check out these poses for a better night's rest. Thanks to Strongfigure Ambassador Steph Kinzer and Kaylie Dao for the photos and descriptions!

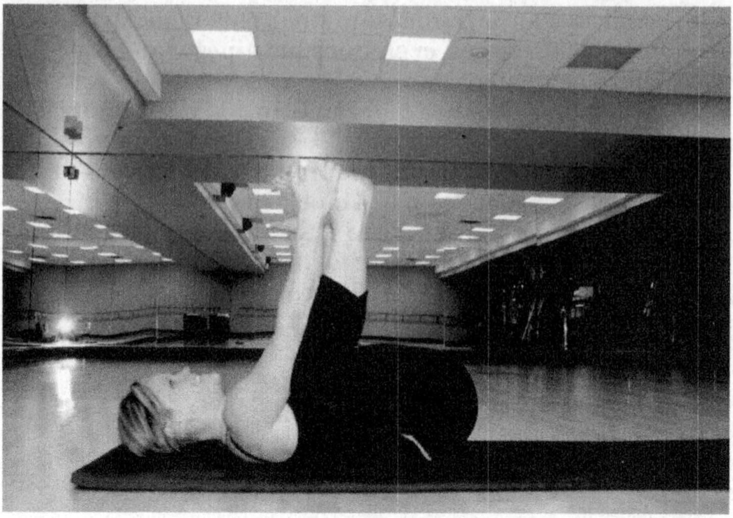

Happy Baby. Laying on your back, hold onto the outsides of your feet and gently pull down on your legs. You want your shins and forearms as vertical as possible. This is also good for lower back pain. Hold for 10 deep breaths, I dare you NOT to smile while holding this.

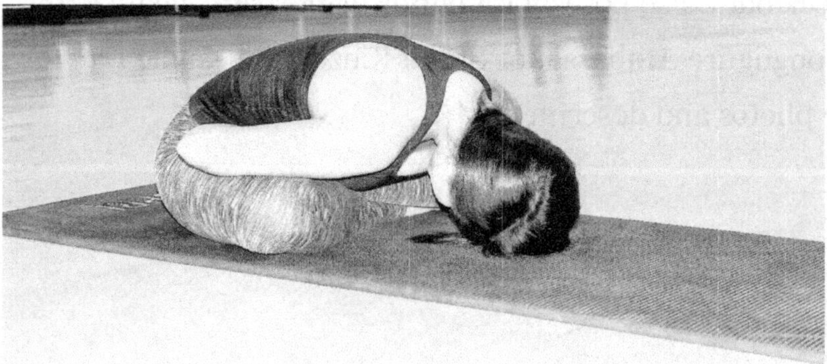

Seated forward Bend: Starting in cross-legged position, hinge forward at your hips and slowly lower your forehead to the floor. To help your head reach, sit on a blanket or pillow. A variation is to keep your legs straight out in front of you and fold over them, grabbing your legs or feet. Relax your face and neck. Give yourself a calf/foot massage for a bonus. Hold for 10 breaths.

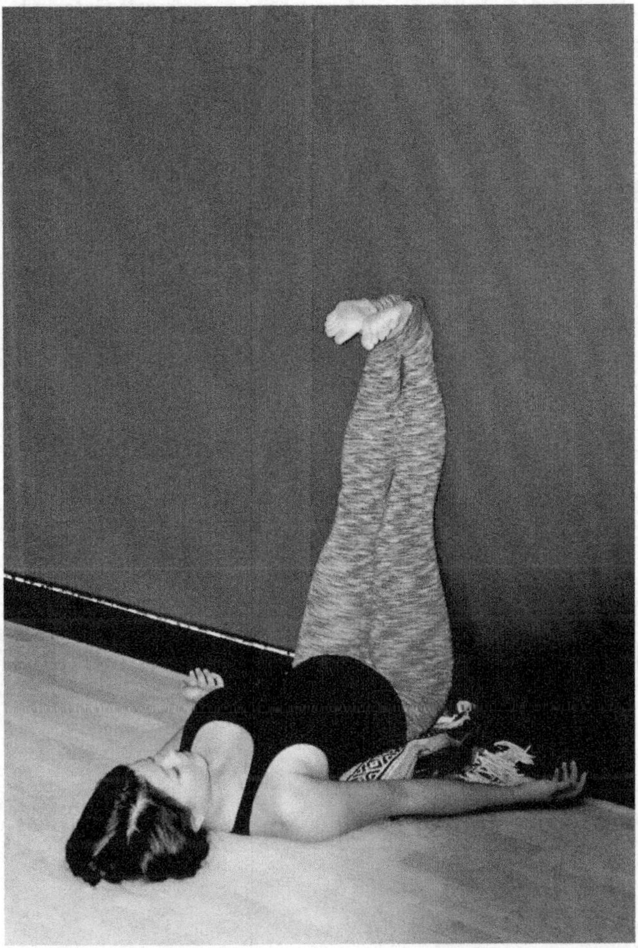

Legs up wall (or headboard). Lay down with your legs up against the wall (or bed) as close as you can get your booty while being comfortable. Place a blanket under your hips/butt for extra comfort and an inversion. Hold your legs up against the wall for up to 5 minutes. This move is great for dealing with edema in your ankles/legs, so I tend to use it when I'm traveling and get swollen feet/ankles. Important to note this pose should not be done if pregnant.

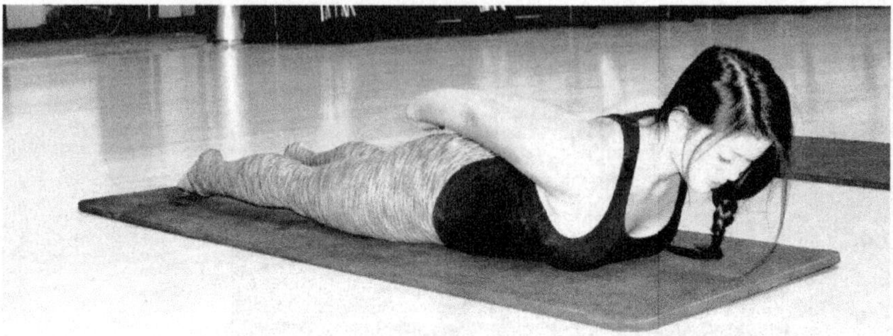

Locust Pose. Starting in a plank position, lower yourself down to your belly. Clasp hands behind your back (or hold them behind you if more comfortable). Keeping tops of your feet pressing against the floor, lift chest, head and arms while looking forward. Hold for up to one minute and repeat 5 times.

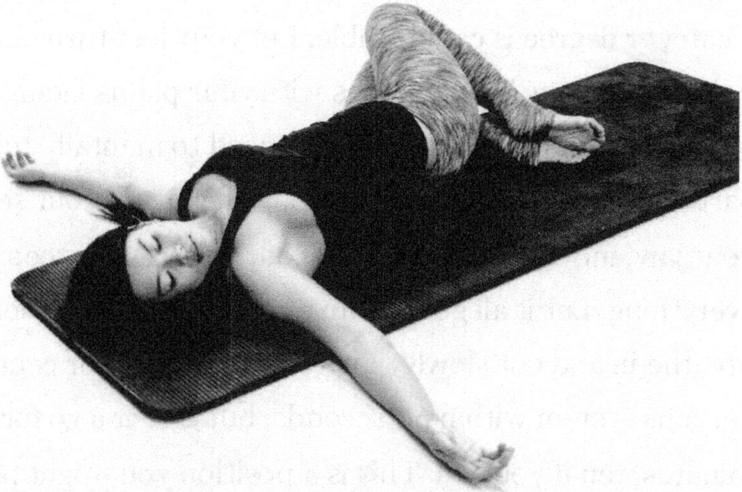

Supine Twist. Lay on your back (hold your arms out in a T-shape if you have the space) keeping knees together and legs bent, let both legs fall to the left side while you look to the right. Hold this for 10 breath cycles to release anxiousness, then switch sides. Twists are great for cleansing your organs also, (your liver) if maybe you aren't sleeping because you had too much wine? It could happen.

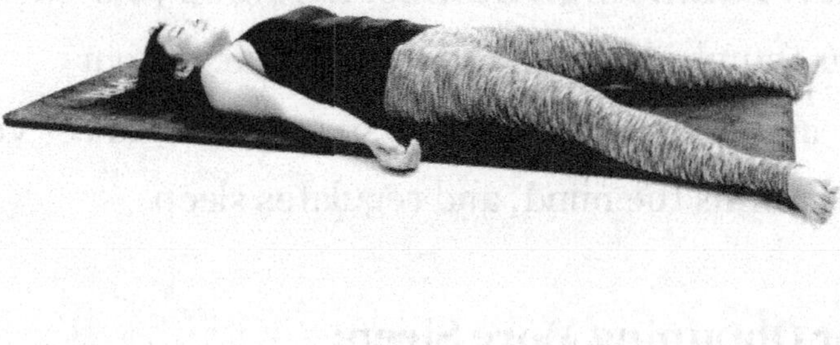

Corpse Pose. This is a fabulous pose to end with. Laying on your back, open your legs to wider than hip width, to whatever degree is comfortable. Let your feet turn out. Relax your arms by your sides with your palms facing up. Stop here and just breathe. If you need to mentally tell each part of your body to relax first you can start at your scalp, your jaw, move to your elbows, your knees, your toes, everything. Let it all go with an exhale breath and then just breathe in and out slowly. This pose relaxes your central nervous system within 60 seconds, but give it a go for a few minutes, ten if you can. This is a position you might pass out in; enjoy every nano second of it.

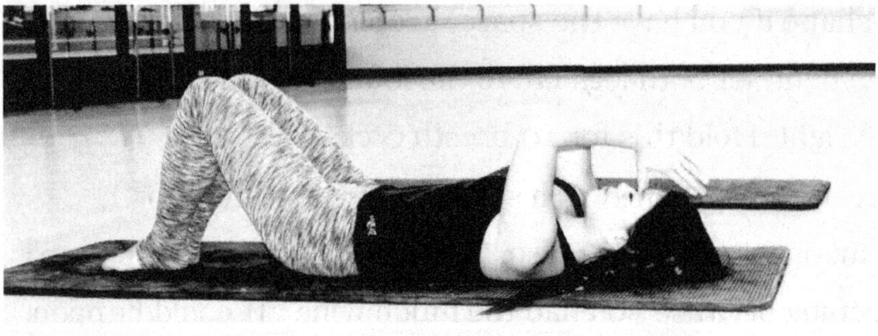

Hormonal Balancing Thumbs. Laying on your back, bring your thumbs to touch the space between your eyebrows and press with light pressure. This balances your hormones, calms the mind, and regulates sleep.

Steps for Obtaining More Sleep:

Assess Your Sleep

Use Dr. Gordon's checklist to assess your sleep:

1. Are you sleeping 8-9 hours a night?
2. Are at least 4-5 hours deep sleep?
3. Do you remember some of your dreams?
4. Do you wake feeling refreshed?

If you answered "No" to any of the above questions then continue to step two.

Step Two: Create a personal sleep hygiene plan.

It is best to create a plan that will best fit your lifestyle and your needs, but here are some things to consider in your plan.

- Avoid coffee or caffeinated beverages 6-8 hours before bedtime.
- Limit alcohol consumption to two to three beverages a day and avoid alcohol two to three hours before bedtime.
- Establish your bedroom as a sleep center.
- Make sure it is dark and quiet.
- Make sure you limit the activities you do in your bedroom to sleep so that your brain begins to connect the room with sleep.
- Keep the temperature cool and well ventilated.

- Establish a pre-sleep routine of 15-30 minutes to prepare your brain for sleep.

During this time consider the following:

- Avoid blue light from TVs, smart phone screens, and computer screens. Blue light blocks the production of melatonin. (Consider using blue-blocking sunglasses)
- Avoid light. Darkness will help the body to produce melatonin.
- Consider implementing a yoga, meditation, or stretch and relax routine. Never underestimate the power of yoga. Yoga has a plethora of benefits, such as digestion, improving blood flow, balancing hormones, increased flexibility, and muscle strengthening.
- Avoid reading materials that will spark too much thought production.
- Establish a consistent schedule for sleep time and wake time. It is best to always sleep and always rise within an hour of your established sleep schedule. If you plan to wake at 6am every morning then on the weekends you need to wake no later than 7am. The body will sleep best when part of a consistent schedule.
- In the morning take vitamin D and eight ounces of water. Vitamin D along with natural light will help you in so many ways, one of which is a better night's sleep.

Many people don't automatically connect energy and time management to health. You see, if you're missing out on sleep (see previous chapter); you're likely running behind on a day-to-day basis. And good sleep or not, sometimes many of us find ourselves lacking the energy we need to do things like exercise, play with the kids, even run errands after work. Energy balance and time management are skills needed for a healthy lifestyle and for obtaining overall confidence and happiness. Having more energy and learning to manage your time better also works to reduce stress--a leading killer in this country--which we'll tackle in the next chapter.

It's imperative you create your own energy and manage your time wisely. Your health is dependent on this!

Have you ever heard someone say, "I'm too tired to go to the gym," and another person responds, "But exercise gives you energy!"? And the first person says, "but how am I supposed to exercise if I don't have the energy in the first place?" ...and the conversation goes round and round.

Exercise does increase one's energy levels. And like we said in earlier in this book, sometimes the hardest part about exercise is just convincing yourself to start. That's why we asked you dig deep and find your "WHY" at the beginning of the book. If you have a "WHY," you have motivation. This motivation will get you moving.

But there are other ways that you can increase your energy without solely relying on exercise. Food actually provides us with a LOT of energy. I mean, isn't that its purpose anyway?

On the flip side, food can also zap our energy. Have you ever sat down after a big meal--Thanksgiving for example--and you found yourself incredibly sleepy within 20 minutes?

When we fill up on too much food or the wrong kinds of food, our bodies just get exhausted. Between the insulin spikes, the digestive system working overboard, and all that food just sitting in our guts...it's no wonder we take a long nap in front of the TV.

We have to stop looking at food as glorious morsels of scrumptiousness and start thinking of food as fuel for our lifestyle.

You are a Ferrari. Are you going to fill yourself up on cheap gasoline? Are you going to stuff your tank so full of that same cheap gas that it starts to spill out of the top? Of course not! You put the right kind of fuel in the right car so that it runs efficiently. You don't overload it and you don't let it run out either. You take care of the nice things you own, right?

Why wouldn't you take care of yourself? You can get the same kind of fueling results all from eating the right kinds and the right amounts of food.

Now, what foods will you choose in order to make up those quantities? Hopefully, energy-boosting ones.

- Water is a key energy-boosting nutrient which we discussed early in Chapter One. Your body is made up of 60-70% water. If you're dehydrated, nothing is working efficiently, and your energy will be considerably less. HYDRATE, HYDRATE, HYDRATE!
- Eating smaller portions of high quality unprocessed foods--especially vegetables--help sustain daily energy. Foods such as spinach, beans, almonds, apples, salmon, eggs, sweet potatoes, brown rice, beets, broccoli, cauliflower, celery, cucumbers, kale, onions, peas, peppers, bananas, berries, melons, lemons, peaches, and pears all provide energy to help boost your body's natural health and daily activity.

When you start sleeping more and you've started to take care of your body through proper nutrition and exercise, your energy is going to soar. And when your energy soars, you have a lot of time in your day to accomplish the things you want and need to do!

But even if you have the world's best energy, knowing how to properly manage your time is a skill that takes a lot of practice. Figuring out how to best manage the business of life can be overwhelming and cause too much stress. And as you'll see in the next chapter, stress is NOT healthy. Being able to manage yourself creates confidence in all that you do. So how do you manage every last detail of your ultra-busy life?

Eliminate, Produce, and Become Efficient.

- Start focusing your time on the tasks that increase your output. For example: scrolling through Twitter probably doesn't increase the productivity of your day; however, making a to-do list would. Start eliminating distractions.
- Delegate tasks that others can help you with. Can your kids fold the laundry for you? Can a co-worker help you with a project? If someone can do the work at least 75% as well as you can, employ his or her assistance.

- Set time limits on your tasks and give yourself deadlines. Each day, write down your "To-Dos" and give yourself time limits and deadlines. You may have a week to get something done, but you can block out one hour each day to work on the project. That's ALL you do during that hour.
- You can also map out your plans. If you know the end goal of a task or project, why not map out all the steps you need to take to reach the finish? This could be done with any project or any goal. Make a plan and attack it with confidence.
- Ever heard of the Pomodoro technique? This is a time management technique in which you work on one activity for 25 minutes, take a 5 minute break, then work on another activity for 25 minutes, etc. There's even a Pomodoro App that helps you with timing and tasks!
- Block out interference and distractions. Personally, I had to turn off ALL my phone notifications so that I could be more productive with my day. You may have to shut a door, turn your phone on silent, close out your email. Whatever it is, block it.
- Don't multi-task. Our brains cannot function on more than one task at a time, and trying to multi-task makes us slower. Sure...you think you're good at it...until you forgot to finish a project or you lost some information, or you ended up in the kitchen without remembering why you walked in there in the first place.... You've got to be fully present in all that you do so you can be as efficient as possible.
- STOP procrastinating. If it has to be done, do it. By accomplishing the tasks you must do, you build your confidence with each completion. Give yourself a strict deadline, schedule the time to work on it, and get it DONE.
- Make a list of things to STOP working on. Did you know that Steve Jobs said that Apple became the leading

technology company because of all the projects they said "NO" to? So stop working on things that don't matter and become completely clear, convinced, and sold on the goals that you are trying to achieve.

- Introduce yourself to a morning routine that will set the stage for your entire day. An appropriate morning routine can get you out of bed excited and eager for your day. A great waking start to your day means automatic productivity, more time, and better energy. Plus it's amazing for your health. Later in this book we will show you how to create a morning routine.

Learning how to manage your time gives you the energy you need to focus on what's important in your life. The two go hand-in-hand. It's almost impossible to have one without the other. And when you learn how to give yourself the energy you need--whether it's through sleep, nutrition, hydration, time management, exercise, or hopefully a combination of them all--your health not only benefits but your happiness and confidence account thrives.

One practical time saving, energy enhancing activity that's great for every person is FOOD PREP.

The most health conscious people you'll ever meet have some sort of food prep method they practice. Whether it's monthly bulk shopping and stuffing the freezer with chicken breasts and broccoli, or it's weekly meals made for the family; food prepping saves time, money, and energy.

Food prep is not easy but it is perhaps the single greatest skill you can acquire in meeting your health and nutrition goals. Here are some tips to help you get started in your food prep journey:

- Start by prepping one meal for the week: lunch. Make a quick grocery list and go to the store for the items you need.
- Prep all of your lunches for the week. Choose a time over the weekend when no one else will be in your kitchen. Grab five appropriate sized containers and measure out your portions to meet your daily calorie/macronutrient goals. If you've got a family, can everyone eat the same thing for lunch? See if the kids can help out! What a great way to bring the family together, teach healthy habits, and get the kids excited about their lunches!
- The next weekend, food prep all of your lunches *and* all of your snacks for the week.
- In weekend three, food prep all of your lunches, all of your snacks, and two dinners.
- By week four you are starting to become an expert! Prep all of your lunches, all of your snacks and 4-5 dinners.

Obviously, if you're prepping for a whole family, things will take time. You're just going to have to experiment, try different recipes, and hopefully those in the family can help you! Can you freeze some of the meals? Can you use a crockpot for easy dinners? Make a breakfast casserole that feeds four? I like to keep food simple: clean, healthy, and quick to prepare. We are living in much too busy of a world to always be bogged down with cooking!

One of the most frustrating "meals" to prep is a healthy snack. If you've got kids, if your metabolism is high functioning, if you need pre-workout food, or if you just need to get in more calories, you're going to want a snack. And there's nothing wrong with that. But finding quick and easy healthy snacks is sometimes much harder than it seems it should be. Luckily, there's Pinterest (https://www.pinterest.com/stephaniejwimer/better-snack-choices/) for recipes on anything you are looking for. But if you don't have Pinterest or you just want a quick list of easy foods, here's a list of our favorites:

- Snow pea pods and your favorite hummus
- Hardboiled eggs with a condiment (I like mustard)
- Cottage cheese (which mixes well with fruits, olives, cucumbers, cherry tomatoes, really whatever you enjoy…)
- Natural peanut butter and celery
- Deli roast beef* and horseradish
- Plain Greek yogurt with your favorite curry spices
- Plain Greek yogurt mixed with a ripe, mashed avocado, with Greek seasonings, onion powder, paprika makes an amazing veggie dip
- Wrap some jicama (Mexican turnip) in deli ham*
- Freeze a banana-almond milk-kale smoothie in ice trays.
- Frozen grapes

- Make your own yogurt parfait with plain Greek yogurt and fresh berries
- Ricotta cheese and strawberries
- Homemade guacamole with endive leaves as dippers
- Tomatoes and goat cheese (our farmer's market has the best goat cheese in a variety of types and flavors)
- Celery sticks with plain hummus and Kalamata olives
- Carrots with a chipotle yogurt sauce (mix 1 tsp chipotles in adobo sauce with ½ cup plain yogurt)
- Sliced cucumbers with Greek seasoning
- Seasonal fruit such as blood oranges (use sparingly since often high in sugar)
- Pickles, jalapenos, and low fat mozzarella (this one might sound strange but it is one of my favorites)
- Snap peas with plain yogurt and Old Bay seasoning.
- Sea salt mixed nuts (can be high calorie so make sure you keep counts to fit within your daily caloric goals)

*Deli meats are quick and easy but should be used sparingly since they are processed meats and often have sulfites. If you do eat foods high in sulfites, eat foods high in molybdenum, such as lima beans. Lima beans help detoxify sulfites.

Understanding that life needs organization is a key factor in your overall health. Figuring out how to plan your meals so that you can get to the gym after work for example, will automatically save you time, give you more energy, and boost your health. This can work in any area of life.

When you have energy and time, your health improves. Your lifestyle improves. Your family health and happiness improves. Imagine how your family would feel if you suddenly had more time to spend with them? If you had the energy to take family adventures? Health isn't just about cutting cupcakes out of your life. It's about creating the time and energy needed to live your life the way it was meant to be lived. On YOUR terms, YOUR way.

Start Planning Your Week Now:

1. One day each week (I typically choose a weekend), plan out your week: what are your top priorities that you must accomplish, no matter what? For me this is family, work, gym, food prep, any other meetings or events.
2. Next, plan out up to three goals you have for the week. One can be a work goal, one could be a life goal, and the other could be a family goal. I typically plan business goals--such as "complete such and such chapter of this book" or "edit chapter ....of ...." Or a personal goal that I want to accomplish for the week.
3. Schedule a day and time to plan your meals, make a list, go grocery shopping, and food

prep. You may not do all these on the same day, but start getting in the habit of scheduling when you will do these.

4. Schedule your exercise time.
5. Create a morning routine.
6. STICK to your schedule. Accomplishing what you say you will accomplish will automatically boost your confidence and do wonders for your self-esteem. If you say you will, and you do, you've already set yourself up for success for the next time that you need to accomplish something important.

"Stress is the number one killer of people worldwide. There is nothing more damaging to your body, your mind, and your emotions, than stress." –Paul Chek

Stress can fall into three different categories and it might be the primary reason you are not achieving the health and fitness results you desire.

The 3 categories of stress:

- **Physical** examples include physical pain, use of medicines and/or drugs, and current or unresolved injuries.
- **Emotional** examples include hormonal imbalances, mood problems, energy highs and lows.
- **Mental** examples include toxic relationships with people, spiritual problems*

*many consider spirituality-related stressors to be a separate category

All categories of stress affect your body. They all add up together and can form quite a lot of unhealthy tension within. Your boss, your significant other, your sick pet or child, your workload...all of these add to your stress and they all negatively affect your health.

Physiologically speaking, the cell does not care about the source of your stress. Stress of a divorce, stress of drug use, and stress of an injury all affect your body at the cellular level the same. Each stressor produces a response in the body that is biochemically identical.

When the body has too much stress it can lead to chronic fatigue, disease, and even death.

Homeostasis

Not all stress is bad. Stress is a natural physiological function that helps us to grow and be stronger. If we were to sit on a couch all day and watch TV we might have very little stress but eventually our body would become weak and we would deteriorate into a very unhealthy being.

But too much stress can also lead to poor health. And because all stress is equal at the cellular level, when you do not fix the stresses in your work and your relationships, adding physical stresses could cause your body to breakdown from too much stress.

To be fully healthy we need to balance our life in a state of homeostasis.

Are You Imbalanced?

Every individual has to balance his or her own life to live in a homeostatic state. For most people, exercise will help with this balance. However, for some people it could potentially be adding to an imbalance.

Symptoms of Stress and Imbalance

1. Behavioral Symptoms: sleeping too much or not enough, eating too much or not enough, isolating yourself from others, drug and alcohol use

2. Emotional Symptoms: mood swings, irritability, unable to relax, feeling overwhelmed, loneliness

3. Cognitive Symptoms: unable to concentrate, anxiousness, worry, poor judgement, memory problems

4. Physical Symptoms: pain, sickness, digestive problems, low libido

If you are showing these symptoms then there is a good chance you are in a state of imbalance.

Manage Your Stress Now:

Step 1: Is this picture moving?

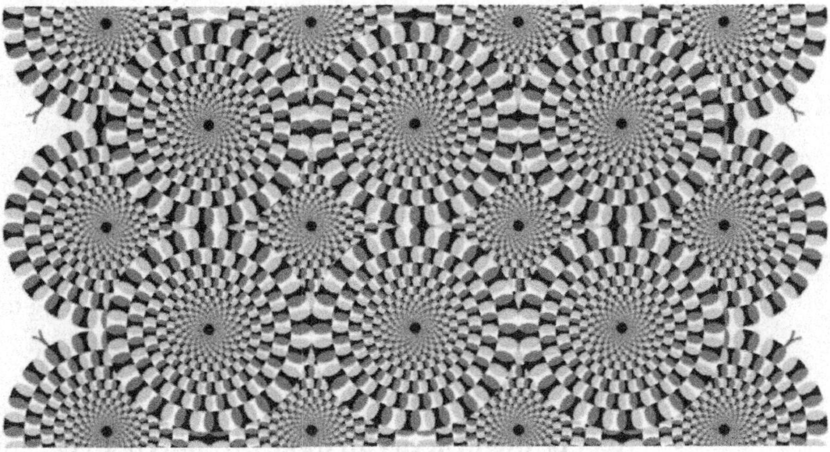

Some scientists use pictures like this to determine physiological stress levels. People with high amounts of stress will see movement in the picture and people with low stress levels will see a still picture.

Take a look at the stressors in your life and analyze what can you do to limit the amount of stress they add to your being.

How Can I Better Balance My Life?

First we need to look at what we can control:

- **Avoid unnecessary stress.** Many of us can improve our life today by simply getting rid of certain areas of our life that are causing stress. If it is possible to avoid the stressor, then eliminate it from your life. Not all stress can be avoided, but by avoiding people and situations that produce stress, and by learning how to distinguish between the things in life you must do from the things in life you feel you should do; you can eliminate many of your daily stressors.
- **Assertion**. If you can't avoid a stressful situation, try to alter it. Be assertive and deal with problems. Do NOT let problems build up or fester. And be willing to compromise and problem-solve a way to peacefully resolve the conflicts in your life.
- **Accept the things you have no control over.** You can only worry about the things that you can change. And always look at the big picture—in the scope of your life does this stressor really matter? There will always be stressors in life that you can't fix or eliminate. Accepting these stressors will help you to balance your life.

Next we need to improve our physical health to better manage our stressors.

- **Relaxation.** Activities like yoga, meditation, prayer, and deep breathing activate the body's relaxation response. By setting aside a time in our day to relax, we counterbalance the stresses in our life.
- **Exercise.** Physical activity can help minimize the negative effects of stress.

- **A combination of meditation and exercise works wonders.** A study at Rutgers University showed that individuals suffering from depression who practiced meditation for 30 minutes followed by aerobic exercise for 30 minutes, acquired new cognitive skills that helped them process information and reduce the overwhelming recollection of memories from the past.
- **Nutrition.** Eating a nutrient rich diet can minimize the negative effects of stress. Also, toxins such as sugar, alcohol, and most preservatives will increase your body's stress levels.
- **Sleep.** High quality sleep of 8-9 hours a night will limit the negative effects of too much stress. When sleeping your body is rebuilding itself for the next day. During quality sleep, you return to homeostasis.
- **Create a morning routine.** (See below)

Do Mornings Better

One of the BEST ways to reduce and manage stress is to learn how to become a morning person OR *revamp* your current morning routine.

Studies are now showing that it might not be as important *how much* you sleep, but *when* you're sleeping. A recent study at Aachen University conducted 59 brain scans, and of those who were early risers, the morning crew had significantly more white matter in the brain--the fatty tissue that facilitates communication among nerve cells. In other words, morning people are more likely to be creative, productive, and have higher cognitive function.

On the flip side, studies by the American Academy of Sleep Medicine have shown that those who sleep late are more likely to eat unhealthy foods and become dependent on alcohol and tobacco. They may even be more prone to depression, anxiety, and other mental illnesses.

You Need a Routine.

The best way to get yourself up in the morning is to figure out a way to get excited about the morning. Then create a morning routine. This may be the hardest part of your wellness challenge, but turning yourself into a morning person is just as great for your health as eating well and exercising. And take note--not only can you make exercising a part of your morning routine, but a morning exerciser is much less likely to blow off workouts.

1. If your brain likes to spin at night and keep you awake, start by making a to-do list for the next day.
2. Figure out what's going to excite you in the morning. A big cup of coffee? Tea? Having time to make a real breakfast? Reading a chapter in your current favorite book? Doing some Pilates or taking a walk with the dog? Give yourself something to look forward to about the morning.

3. Start with small increments and slowly start going to bed a little earlier each night. If you want to get up 30 minutes earlier to begin your day, you only need to go to bed 30 minutes earlier. Start with five or ten minute increments and getting to bed earlier will be a piece of cake.
4. Turn off your blue lights--phone, tv, iPad, etc., and turn your technology to airplane mode. Did you know that your phones and other smart devices are constantly searching for signals and this can interfere with your sleep? So get your phones on airplane mode and better yet, put them across the room (if you use them for an alarm) or in a different room.
5. Build your perfect morning routine.

I learned how to build a morning routine from Hal Elrod's ***Miracle Morning*** book. This book is one of the best books I've read for my health. Erik and I now wake up 30-60 minutes earlier than normal (even on weekends!) in order to plan our days and focus on our health. Creating a morning routine has brought back more energy to our days, reduced our stress, helped our management skills, and leaves us feeling accomplished and successful--all attributes to better total body health.

So Hal has created these simple morning "Life SAVERS" that start his day and have been starting the days for millions of people worldwide. His life savers stand for **Silence** (meditation or guided thought), **Affirmations** (telling yourself what you want to believe about yourself, your life, your day), **Visualization** (seeing yourself each and every day being successful at whatever it is you are trying to do) **Exercise** (even if it's just a 15 minute stretching or mobility routine, a quick walk through the neighborhood, or a few push-ups and sit-ups), **READING** (even if it's just a paragraph) and **Scribing** (writing out your thoughts, making a list, or jotting down your goals for the day).

People who take anywhere from 15 minutes to an hour each morning to incorporate these life savers into their routines will undoubtedly become more productive and increase their health, energy, and happiness.

But how do you go from waking up at 7am all the way to 6am without struggle?

You don't. You start with 10-15 minute increments. If you typically wake up at 7, set your alarm for 6:45 and make sure you have to get out of bed to reach the alarm. DO NOT get back in bed. Drink water. Brush your teeth. Put clothes on–whatever you have to do.

The rest is up to you: you're awake and out of bed!

Our suggestions for creating a morning routine follow closely to Hal's. After all, this stuff has a proven success rate.

It doesn't matter what order you use when you create your routine, just do what feels right for you. Here's what Erik and I like to do.

- Have some coffee and sit in silence. You can meditate if you want, or simply sit and breathe, or you can focus on a positive word or phrase you'd like to become better with in your life. Words like "confidence," "patience," "gratitude," etc., are easy words to focus on.
- Create a vision board and look at your board for a few minutes. What are your goals? Your "whys"? Meaning, why is this important to you? What do you want to accomplish and what's your end goal? Put it on the board and focus on your vision.

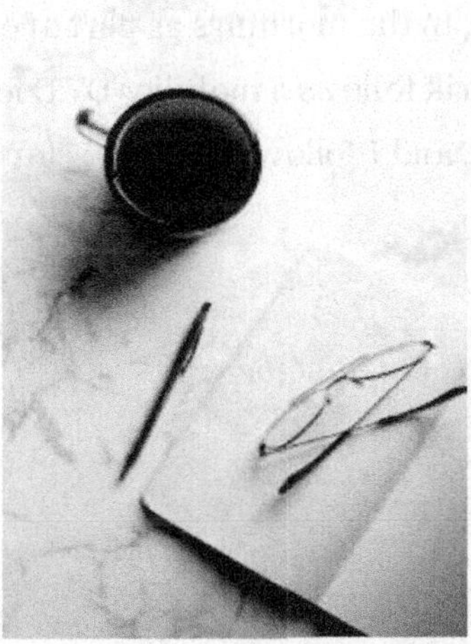

- Read a chapter (or just a couple pages) from a book: you can read personal growth books (when you work on you, everything else gets better), you can read business-related books for work, spiritual books, or just for fun fiction novels or magazines. Try to do something good for yourself here and flipping through the internet to catch up on social media doesn't count!

- Write down your to-do list, your weekly goals, your new affirmation or positive phrase, or just journal something. Make a plan for your day, write out a menu, tackle personal goals and business ideas, whatever you want to write! It doesn't–and shouldn't be–long. It only needs to be long enough to get you thinking and your brain feeling confident about the day ahead.
- Move. Thousands of people have actually lost weight and gotten their health back in order just from adding in a good 10-20 minutes of exercise into their morning routine. You don't have to work out for an hour, you just have to do something good for your body. You can stretch, follow a yoga or other fitness DVD, take your dog for a walk, go for a few sprints around the block–whatever it is, it's going to improve your health. Since Erik and I typically workout later in the day, in the mornings as part of our routine, Erik follows a mobility DVD for his tight back, and I follow ROMWOD for total body mobility.

Try romwod for free here:
https://romwod.com/members/aff/go/strongfigure

Dealing with stress is largely an issue every individual needs to address in their own life, through their own solutions. If stress is not managed it will eventually lead to sickness and death. You cannot turn your health around until you learn how to manage your stress.

What do you say? Can you incorporate some time in your morning to create a game plan for starting your day on the right foot? Can you make it so that you go to bed early enough to wake up a bit earlier? 10 minutes? 20? 30? An hour? Studies show that if you take the time to wake up and map out your day with a list, take time to say or write down your positive affirmations about yourself, educate yourself through a few minutes of reading, and performing roughly 10 or so minutes of exercise or stretching, it's impossible to NOT have a successful, productive, positive day.

Take a little time to investigate, on your own, the power of creating your own miracle morning. And since reading should be a part of your morning, check out Hal's book, Miracle Morning. *(We aren't affiliated with Hal or his book. We're just practitioners and believers.)* The power you have to rewire your brain, praise yourself for your accomplishments, write out some affirmations and keep a journal of your goals and successes, educate yourself on better mindful practices, and learn from your mistakes will take your health further than any plan of just "diet and exercise."

Other steps you can take to start immediately reducing your stress:

Following the steps outlined in the earlier chapters will greatly lower your stress levels. Research shows that properly addressing all of the other essential keys to health and fitness: sleep, nutrition, exercise, energy, time management, and hydration, will help reduce stress. In addition to working on improving ALL areas of wellness, let's take a closer look at reducing stress.

Step One: Eliminate or reduce the toxins

Toxins are a tremendous source of stress on the body. Our recommendation is to eliminate all narcotics and tobacco from your life. We also recommend a reduction in the amount of alcohol and sugar you consume, especially if you have other forms of stress affecting your life.

Step Two: Take a daily morning walk

Walking in the morning can benefit your health and fitness in so many ways. Research shows that a 10-15 minute walk, while bouncing a ball periodically, is shown to be more effective at reducing stress and anxiety than Prozac and other anti-anxiety medicines.

Step Three: Meditate

Research also shows that spending a few minutes throughout the day in meditation can restore your calm and inner peace and have tremendous health benefits. There are so many ways people are able to meditate: prayer, yoga, tai chi, mantra meditation, guided meditation. There are even free apps you can download such as "Guided Mind" which will help you reduce your stress. Find what works for you. Pick up a recommended book on meditation and give it a try. If a few minutes of mindfulness can reduce all that stress in your life, what do you have to lose?

Step Four: If all else fails start a journal

Try steps 1-3 first and if you still feel you need help coping with and reducing your stress levels then why not give journaling a try. Many report that keeping a stress journal has allowed them to greatly reduce their anxiety.

In your journal:

- Identify the recurring stressors that affect your life and how you deal with them.
- Try different coping methods to remedy these regular stressors and report how each of them makes you feel.
- Use this journal whenever you feel stressed and self-assess the solutions that work best for you.

Step 5: Work on your own personal growth and emotional development

Changing your mental attitude about yourself is going to be the toughest and possibly most important step in your quest for a healthier life and for *positive* change.

While you can spend *years* learning about nutrition, macro and micro nutrients, Paleo diets, yoga, strength training, conditioning workouts, stretching and mobility, how to food prep, or even how order out and not screw up your diet when hanging with your friends; sitting around and comparing yourself to every fitness figure on Instagram and Pinterest, and beating yourself up every time you do something "wrong" is going to lead you nowhere other than a dark place consumed with self-abuse, ridicule, and depression.

"I screwed up again--I'm such a loser."
"I have no willpower. I should just quit."

"I'll never have the body I want."
"I hate my ________ (fill in the blank)."

Sound like you?

Your attitude is going to be the number one key to your new journey in a life filled with good health. Remember we discussed this in the introduction. If you can't control your mindset, you'll never reach your goals. Know that it's ok to make mistakes. We all understand this. And we all teach our children, our friends, that when we make mistakes, we learn from them and keep going. Why should your health be any different? It's ok to make errors. But it's not ok to consistently verbally abuse yourself, shatter your own self-esteem, and hate your body. It's not ok to feel like a failure.

By convincing yourself that you are doing your very best at that moment in time and you love who you are in this journey--right where you are--then you are sending positive vibes to your inner conscious. And guess what? Those triggers will start working for you even when you are unaware. It will also be much *much* easier to reach your goals when your mind is positive and you enjoy who you are.

When you wake up in the morning and look in the mirror and tell yourself that you love what you see (whether you do or you don't), your brain will start to make the connections you need to start appreciating all that you are doing for yourself each and every day to make yourself the best you that you are currently searching for. Whether you believe it or not, start now, telling yourself that you love who you are. Even if you have to pick one body part or characteristic that you love, focus on it and be happy.

"Before success comes in any man's life, he is sure to meet with much temporary defeat, and, perhaps, some failure. When defeat overtakes a man, the easiest and most logical thing to do is to quit. That is exactly what the majority of men do. More than five hundred of the most successful men this country has ever known told the author their greatest success came just one step beyond the point at which defeat had overtaken them." -- Napoleon Hill, Think and Grow Rich

You might want to quit. But how do you know if the day your life turns around isn't just right around the corner?

In Richard O'Connor's book about rewiring the brain, he wrote

"Neuroscientists know now that bad habits have a physical existence in the structure of the brain; they become the default circuits when we are faced with temptation."

Your brain is like a muscle and you are exercising that muscle daily. And if you consciously tell yourself every day that you love your body, you are strong, you are powerful--

anything you want to believe about yourself--sooner or later your inner conscious is going to believe it without you telling it. The power of thought, meditation, personal affirmations, and self-love may be the single best exercises you can do for yourself.

Think about it this way: if you worked on push-ups every single day for a year, do you think you would be better at push-ups 365 days later? How could you not? The brain works the same way. Day one might be tough to love yourself for who you are right now. Day 10 may be even worse because you had a setback on day nine. Day 365? You'll love yourself in no time.

"You are the master of your destiny. You can influence, direct and control your own environment. You can make your life what you want it to be." Napoleon Hill, Think and Grow Rich

Speaking of Setbacks

Richard O'Connor's book *Rewire Your Brain to Break Bad Habits* outlined what happened during an experiment on food choice related to the "I screwed up" attitude of dieters.

Two groups of dieters were given a dessert. Group A was given a fruit and yogurt bowl that added up to about 500+

calories. Group B was given a small bowl of ice cream that came to about 250 calories. Both groups were told how many calories were in the bowl.

Guess what happened? Group A, the group who ate the healthier fruit and yogurt bowl, ate less throughout the rest of the day. The group who ate the ice cream said, 'screw it,' and ate more the rest of the day AND made worse decisions when it came to what they ate--all because they felt as if they "screwed up" by having ice cream.

If Group B had just continued to make healthy decisions after the ice cream, they wouldn't have blown their diets. They wouldn't have had experienced food guilt the next day. They would have stayed the course and continued their progress. But because they had ice cream, even KNOWING they had fewer calories than the fruit and yogurt group, they blew their calorie intake for the whole day! They totally said 'screw it,' even though they were technically ahead of the game – all over a little bowl of ice cream!" Read more from my post here: http://strongfigure.com/battle-guilt-with-your-most-powerful-musde/

How many times have you done this exact same thing in your quest to become healthier? How many times have you thought we actually failed when really you haven't? And how many times have you given up because you stopped believing in your abilities to succeed?

"We have a plastic brain that changes in response to our experience. It bears repeating: The brain doesn't tell us what to do; it is part of a system in which our life experience teaches our brain what to do. So you can practice mindfulness, willpower, overcoming procrastination, and other healthy new skills with the confidence that you are changing your brain. Each day's practice does some good, and if you slip and fall off your diet or exercise program or mindfulness practice, all that you have learned before is not undone; it's still there in your brain waiting for you to get back in the saddle." Rewire: Change Your Brain to Break Bad Habits by Dr. Richard O'Connor.

Step 6: Create Your Own Miracle Morning

Hal's **"Life SAVERS"** have been helping millions of people worldwide establish success each and every day. **Silence, Affirmations, Visualization, Exercise, READING**, and **Scribing** can give you the jump start you need for a better, healthier lifestyle.

Aren't these the same steps for stress reduction and creating a healthier mind?

You can't fix just part of the self. You've got to work on the whole self to have total success. You'll make mistakes. You'll have setbacks. You'll have a bad day, a bad week, heck, you may have a bad year. It doesn't mean that you can't change. And it doesn't mean that you're some sort of failure destined to live unhappily for the rest of your life.

Attitude is everything in your journey. And that's why it is so important to work on becoming mentally strong as well as physically strong. Becoming mentally and emotionally strong may be harder than any weight you ever pick up in the gym. Becoming confident and looking yourself in the mirror every day and appreciating your journey while motivating yourself to continue and visualizing your own end goal, is REALLY hard. That's why it's the most overlooked part of being "healthy" because there's no set workout routine and nutrition plan you put your brain on. You are 100% responsible for reading the books, learning how to love you, and developing your own routine for success: one that works for you and perhaps, no one else.

If you know and realize this from the start, you will have a better chance of pushing through the more challenging days.

The mind is your most powerful muscle and you have the opportunity to exercise it every single day, at any time, in any place. You won't always have control of the food you're given or even your ability to exercise the way you want each day. But you CAN consistently exercise your mind, your will, your thought, and your self-worth.

Improve your brain NOW:

Step one: Start reading! (Or listening to audiobooks while you drive, clean, exercise, etc.) Here's a fantastic list in no particular order:

- *Rewire: Change Your Brain to Break Bad Habits* by Richard O'Connor, PhD
- *Miracle Morning* by Hal Elrod
- *Think and Grow Rich* by Napoleon Hill
- *How to Win Friends and Influence People* by Dale Carnegie
- *How Successful People Think* by John C. Maxwell
- *Undoing Perpetual Stress* by Richard O'Connor, PhD
- *The Organized Mind: Thinking Straight in the Age of Information Overload* by Daniel J. Levitin
- *Rewire Your Brain: Think Your Way to a Better Life* by John B. Arden, PhD
- *Mini Habits: Smaller Habits, Bigger Results* by Stephen Guise
- *The Practicing Mind: Developing Focus and Discipline in Your Life* by Thomas M. Sterner
- *The 7 Habits of Highly Effective People* by Stephen Covey
- *Stumbling on Happiness* by Dan Gilbert
- *A Short Guide to a Happy Life* by Anna Quindlen
- *The Life-Changing Magic of Tidying Up: The Japanese Art of Decluttering and Organizing* by Marie Kondo

- *The Art of Learning: An Inner Journey to Optimal Performance* by Josh Waitzkin
- *Don't Sweat the Small Stuff and It's All Small Stuff: Simple Ways to Keep the Little Things from Taking Over Your Life* by Richard Carlson
- *Who Moved My Cheese? An Amazing Way to Deal with Change in Your Work and in Your Life* by Spencer Johnson and Kenneth Blanchard

Building Your Confidence Account

Gaining confidence and learning to love yourself each and every day is a critical, crucial, and possibly the toughest part of your journey to total body health and wellness.

I can't stress this chapter enough: Confidence and happiness are the peak of the total body wellness pyramid. And when Erik and I wrote the Total Health and Fitness Makeover (the precursor to this book), we didn't even include a chapter on this. I didn't even realize that it existed yet.

All my adult life, I was on a quest to learn how to exercise the BEST way and eat the BEST way. I experimented with so many methods that I couldn't wait to write about all of them--to tell you all my successes, my troubles, my failures, my setbacks. What worked, what didn't. I had no idea when I began my own fitness journey that it would lead here.

I have spent over 10+ years now educating myself in the field of fitness, nutrition, health, and wellness. From senior wellness to children's nutrition, my thirst for knowledge has exceeded any other passions I've had about anything in my lifetime. Getting consumed by the fitness industry, working in the health field, coaching others--it's nothing I ever expected when I started my journey. But when I started looking for guidance so many years ago, I wanted one thing and one thing only: to lose weight.

I began my journey much like anyone else...probably a lot like you. I read a lot of books, went to Weight Watchers meetings, and took group fitness classes at my local gym. One of the first books I read was How to Eat, Move, and Be Healthy by Paul Chek (full URL in references), and it's still one of my favorites! In all that I've read over the years, there are only a small handful of leaders whose words have truly stuck with me; whose teachings really impacted my life and further learning. Paul Chek is one. He caught my attention by saying that too many people will buy expensive cars but won't buy organic produce. Good point, right? He also said, "Sure--organic foods are a bit more expensive, but not as expensive as your hospital bills when your health fails."

Ouch. I read that over ten years ago and never forgot it. I learned so much from Chek. And before you think I'm digressing too much, there's one element to living healthy that Check stressed in his book--and I rolled my eyes to it and moved right along to my next book. That was the part of meditation, spirituality, and happiness.

You may have just rolled your eyes as well. But I wish I had taken that part of the book seriously. I hate to admit it, but it took me too long to realize that my number one goal of losing weight, wasn't going to lead to happiness. Having a *healthy* body (not just a smaller one that looks good), confidence in myself, and doing my very best each day--that is happiness.

I did lose weight. You will too if you follow chapters one and two in this book. But as I lost weight, I wanted more. We always want more, right? I wanted to lose more. I wanted to lift more. I became strong but I wanted to get stronger. I was fit but I wanted six-pack abs. Body fat tests would put me between 17-19% but that was never lean enough. There was always someone who was stronger. Leaner. Better abs. And social media started bringing me down. *"I can't do that. Look like that. Lift like that. Be like that."*

Comparison kills our success. It brings us stress, depression, and sometimes, even binge eating! Comparison kills our health.

The worst thing you can do is compare yourself, your progress, and your journey to someone else.

No matter who you are or where you are in your journey, you've got to understand ONE thing: YOU are YOU. You are doing your best with what you've got every single day. You can't compare yourself to the fitness model on Instagram and you can't compare yourself to the fit mom on Facebook. You are where you are meant to be right now and you have GOT to appreciate your journey. Don't spend your life in a state of *"I hate my thighs."* Spend your life in a state of *"I am strong and I love my body."*

It's a fact that the more positive you are and the more you complement your body, the healthier you will become. The mind is so incredibly powerful. In fact, it is your best tool you have in this journey. I ignored my mind for too long and just like all that I write about--I want you to learn from my mistakes and do the things that work! Building your mindset--just like we started with in the intro--is going to be key to your overall success. Start getting positive about yourself right now and head into this journey with the right attitude.

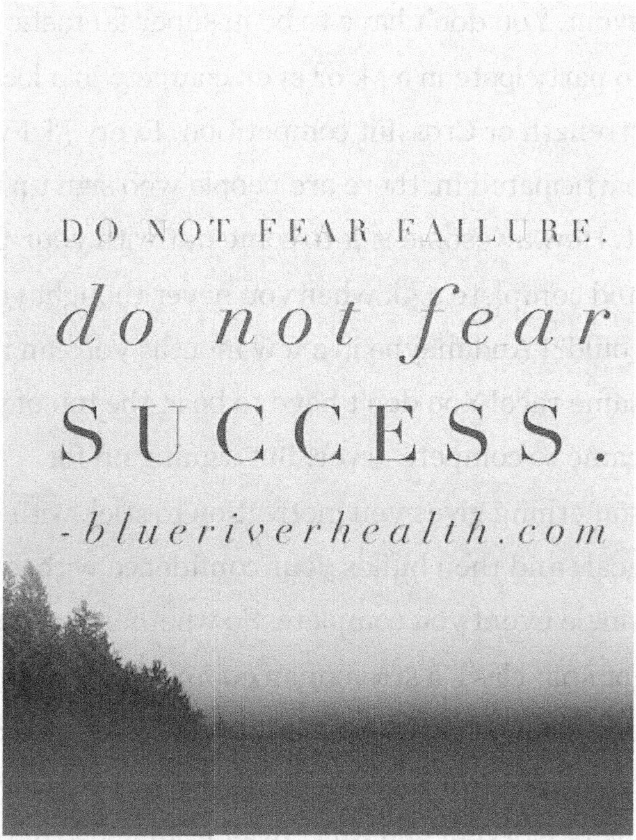

Here's my top 10 list of things you need to start doing RIGHT NOW as you prepare yourself for your new journey to wellness.

1. **Exercise.** We devoted an entire chapter to exercise--why you need to do it and how to do it. But I can't stress enough how much your confidence is going to soar each and every time you commit yourself to a workout. You know what else helps

boost your self-esteem? Signing up for an athletic event. You don't have to be in super fantastic shape to participate in a 5k or even compete in a local strength or CrossFit competition. Every 5k I've participated in, there are people who sign up to walk it. How awesome is it to come out with your friends and complete a 5k when you never thought you could?! And maybe in a few months you can run that same race! You don't have to be at the top of your game to compete--ever. But signing up for something gives you motivation to stick with your goals and then builds your confidence with every single event you complete. So whether you sign up for spin class, a strongman competition, or you just commit yourself to 30 minutes of walking each day--completing your goal will boost your self-esteem and every workout you walk away from will leave you feeling tremendously successful.

2. Think positive, act positive. Do you criticize too quickly? Do you speak negatively without thinking sometimes? I know--many times it's just hard to always act happy. But even if you aren't, you've got to try. If you can smile when you're angry, you won't stay angry for long. If someone ticks you off, put yourself in that person's shoes before you fill your mind with hate. Can you sympathize?

What about when life throws a grenade your way? I struggle with this one too--it's really easy to get angry and stay angry. But Hal Elrod, the Miracle Morning author, said that if there's nothing you can do about the situation or the circumstance, spend five minutes being angry, and then get over it. Find something positive and work towards finding hope or positivity in whatever has been thrown your way. I know it sounds much easier said than done, but Hal came to this conclusion after he had been in a car accident that almost killed him. He was incredibly angry when he awoke in the hospital but he knew he couldn't sit there and just be angry. He couldn't heal any faster by holding onto his anger. Even though doctors thought he wouldn't walk again, he developed an incredibly positive attitude and wasn't just able to walk again, but he competed in marathons. A positive mind, attitude, mental state--it's *everything*.

3. **Kill negativity in your life--your own thoughts, and those who are constantly negative.** Ok, don't kill negative people--even though you may want to sometimes. But seriously,

first and foremost--you DO have to kill the negativity in your head. Just like our positivity tips, if you have a voice that tells you you're fat, you're a loser, you can't run a 5k, you'll never win.....guess what? You won't.

"Optimism is the faith that leads to achievement. Nothing can be done without hope and confidence." Helen Keller.

One of the best books I read, Richard O'Connor's Rewire Your Brain (full URL in references), is full of information about how you can train your brain to think differently. Let me tell you first hand: it's hard. If you've been telling yourself that you hate your hips for 20 years, you can't break your thoughts overnight. In fact, your thoughts are so powerful that they're already ingrained into your subconscious. Remember in the introduction how we talked about always being conscious of your thoughts? It's going to be hard and take a while, but you've got to be in charge of your thoughts. Tell yourself daily that you love your hips and in six months? A year? You will actually love your hips. It sounds silly, but it works. Start loving and complimenting yourself and before long, not only will you become more confident and happier, but because of your confidence, you'll make healthier decisions and start living a healthier life.

It's all tied together. Your mental state is truly going to control your health.

As for people? I know, it's really hard to control negative people in your life. You may work with negative people. You may have negative family members. And you may be a bit more passive than you are aggressive--meaning it may be tough for you to stick up for yourself and tell the negative people to stop being so damn negative! Other than learning how to be more aggressive (in a good way--fighting for your health), one way I've learned to distance myself from negativity is to ignore it. If your co-workers are having a negative conversation, don't join in, even if you want to. If you can walk away, walk away. If you can close your door, close it. If you can't, you can kindly let the person know that you don't enjoy hearing such negativity and you'd rather talk about positive things. You can't always escape it, but you can do your best to be positive and act as a role model for those around you.

Did you know that you act like the five people you spend the most time with? If your top five people are not positive, you may need to rethink your circle. It's tough to walk away from friendships sometimes, but do you really need to poison your mind with toxic relationships? And if you can't walk away, think about being the most positive person you can be and hopefully your attitude can rub off on others.

The same applies for success. If you can hang around the top five successful people you know, you'll be successful. If you hang around the top five richest people you know, you'll increase your wealth. You are who you hang out with. Think about this. If you want to be healthy, fit, successful, and happy--it's time to find those people in your life--seek them out and join their tribe.

4. Get to know yourself, complement yourself, and trust yourself.

Who would have thought I'd have fallen in love with spaghetti squash? Not me. Not until I tried it. When you take the time to try new things, you can't imagine how much you'll end up surprising yourself. I didn't eat very healthy growing up, but I love healthy foods now. I didn't exercise much when I was young but if I had never started, I'd have never found a love for powerlifting and CrossFit. Once I started focusing on "me" I found that I was good at strength training. That's instant confidence! Getting to know myself helped me learn that I didn't have big hips and thighs like I thought I did--I had the ability to build awesome quads! I learned about my body type--someone who could gain both muscle and fat easily if I didn't watch my food intake. The process is about learning, and when you really start to trust both yourself and the process, you'll also start seeing the results. Wake up, take a look in the mirror, and instead of saying "I hate my thighs," say "I have awesome quads and glutes." Instead of saying "I hate my arms," say "I love my biceps!" Get used to complimenting yourself and sooner than later, not only will this positivity become engrained in your subconscious, but you'll also start believing yourself. And when you believe, good things start to happen.

5. Become prepared and follow through.

If you write in your planner that you're going to go to the gym after work, unless an emergency happens, you've got to go to the gym after work. If you tell yourself you're going to the gym three times this week, you've got to go to the gym three times this week. If you want to eat healthy, you can't buy Pop Tarts at the grocery store. You've got to follow through on your plans. Every single time you follow through on something you said you'd do, your confidence builds. Every time you don't follow through on your plans, your confidence dwindles. The more you do for yourself, the bigger your self-esteem. Make plans. Make grocery lists. Prepare your meals in advance. Be consistent with your workouts. The more you follow through with your plans, the bigger your confidence and the better your end results.

6. **Be kinder, and listen. Help others. Volunteer.** The gist of this book is how to focus on you. Complement yourself. Boost your self-esteem, be the best you that you can be. And being a better you also means being a better person. When you stop and truly listen to what another person is saying, you're showing empathy, compassion, and kindness. You're showing that you care about someone else's feelings and that your world doesn't necessarily revolve around your thoughts only. I'm sure you've been in a situation before where you've had a rough day and you needed someone to talk to but the person you chose just didn't seem interested? It's pretty hurtful. Being a kinder person--stopping to listen when no one else does, lending a helping hand, even volunteering your time or services to your community will make you feel accomplished and boost your self-esteem. Even visiting friends and family you haven't seen in a while will do wonders

for your soul. While you work on being the better you, don't forget that that means working on your relationship with others, as well as how you handle others. Patience, kindness, compassion, helpfulness--mastering your ability to be kind and really listen to what others have to say is a trait that not many people have. But once you do? Your esteem will flourish because you have made yourself honest, trustworthy, and kind.

7. **Create small goals, change small habits, and expect success.** I hate clichés, but we all know the famous one is true: *Rome wasn't built in a day*. If you haven't been active or eating healthy for a while now and you decide tomorrow that you're going to exercise five days a week, cut out all sugar, eat six servings of veggies each day, drink a gallon of water every day…….by the end of the week, you'll be exhausted! This is a lifelong journey and I can't stress that enough. Why don't you start with one or two small goals: stop drinking soda and drink more water instead? Walk 30 minutes a day each day. Once you've turned one small goal into a habit, you can then focus on the next goal. Michael Phelps probably didn't start swimming lessons by claiming that his goal was the Olympics. He probably started with smaller goals, smaller competitions, and

eventually grew into a record-breaking Olympic swimmer. You've got to do the same thing with yourself. Maybe creating a morning routine will be your first goal. And once you've made your morning routine your habit, you can then add a few minutes of exercise. Then you add a few servings of veggies. After a while, each small goal turns to habit and habits stick. Once you've changed your unhealthy habits to healthy ones, expect nothing but success, confidence, and the will to tackle any challenge life throws your way.

8. Focus on solutions, get over procrastination. We all know what our problems are: we eat too much or too little, we don't exercise enough, we don't stretch or get enough sleep. We criticize ourselves, we stress over work and relationships, we're tired, lack focus and energy, and we procrastinate by saying *"I'll do better tomorrow."* But this isn't the way we should be thinking. If you know what's wrong, then it's time to focus on solutions. Do you criticize yourself? Praise yourself. Do you eat too much at dinner? Focus on appropriate portion sizes. Are you tired at work? Go to bed 30 minutes earlier. It's time to start focusing on the solutions to your problems--not dwelling on the actual problems. And once you hone in on your solutions and what you need to do, you MUST take immediate action. Saying that you'll start tomorrow just buys yourself more time to slack. How many times have you said "I'll start eating healthy on Monday" and you binge on junk food all weekend? How is this focusing on a solution? It's not helping you; it's hurting you! Procrastination delays progress. Those who are successful take immediate action. And taking control of your problems, tackling them one by one builds your confidence so that you can take on bigger issues as you face them.

9. **Be grateful.** You are not allowed to tear yourself down. You cannot have a bad moment or a bad day and make yourself feel guilty over slipping off the wagon for a brief moment. You are trying your best to take care of yourself and guilt tripping yourself every time you make a mistake isn't going to advance your progress. You're human and we make mistakes. We also learn from them. Be grateful for the journey you're on. Be grateful for what you do for yourself each day and for all that you've learned. You're a better person right now than you were yesterday and you'll be even better tomorrow. You've got to be grateful each and every day for all that you are and all you're doing for yourself. Show compassion to yourself and allow yourself the time

to change and grow. Some days I found myself struggling because I hadn't met the goal that I had intended to meet yet and then I would think to myself--I'm alive and healthy and able to work hard to meet these goals. We can't forget who we are, where we've come from, and how we have been able to meet our goals. Be grateful for each and every day and you will build a solid foundation of hope, happiness, and gratitude that no one can take from you.

10. **Educate yourself.** I think I started off with *Nutrition for Dummies* when I realized I had an interest in learning more about food. More than ten years later, I believe I've read more than 50 books (probably more?) on both exercise and nutrition, and that's not including several classes, courses, certifications, or the daily updated published research and websites I devour in order to stay on top of trends, fads, what works, what doesn't, what science has newly proven, and what has been proven obsolete. You've got to read information. You have to read labels. You have to know why you should lift weights, not just because we told you to do so. You need to try new things, experiment, and hypothesize. Learn from this book but explore further. See what works for you and find out what doesn't. The more

you know about exercise, food, sleep, stress, and your body; the more successful you're going to be. And the more you know and understand, the more confident you'll be in your choices and the game plan you set out for yourself. As adults, we should never stop learning. Our health should be one of our primary focuses as we age, and we need to continue to learn about our bodies, what foods we need, how much sleep we should be getting, how much water we need, and what kind of exercise works best for us. We are all different and I can only provide the basics. It's up to YOU to go out and study: study food, yourself, your environment, your wants, your needs. It's up to YOU to educate yourself and protect your body with the right resources.

And there you have it: six essential steps to help change your life into a much healthier, happier, and more successful YOU. Some steps may be easier than others and for many, all the steps may be pretty tough. That's ok. You can start with one step at a time. Tackle nutrition and hydration first. Then start moving more. Before you know it, getting more sleep and working on your emotional strength will be second nature. Your confidence and self-assurance will begin to flourish and before long, you'll be helping, motivating, and inspiring others to hop on the same wellness path. There's nothing stopping you and no one standing in your way. It's time for you to go out there and REVAMP your health!

Good luck and be sure to join our group on Facebook where you can ask questions and be a part of a bigger movement working to REVAMP health one body at a time!

Resources:

http://www.naturalnews.com.

http://www.womansday.com/food-recipes/food-drinks/g2071/best-foods-for-energy/

http://www.amazon.com/How-Eat-Move-Be-Healthy/dp/1583870067

http://zenhabits.net/25-killer-actions-to-boost-your-self-confidence/

http://www.amazon.com/Rewire-Overcome-Addictions-Self-Destructive-Behavior-ebook/dp/B00FX7UL86/ref=sr_1_1?s=books&ie=UTF8&qid=1458826500&sr=1-1&keywords=rewire+your+brain+to+break+bad+habits

http://www.precisionnutrition.com/problem-with-calorie-counting-calories-in

https://www.crossfitinvictus.com/blog/top-3-supplements-for-a-better-night-of-sleep/

http://www.acidalkalinediet.net/alkaline-foods.php

https://www.sciencedaily.com/releases/2016/02/160210134834.htm

https://foundrmag.com/get-up-early/?inf_contact_key=c34efa05f0bee6dd0a27e660b4894a869436e881bce3a41b2ccb1e8a0802f282

https://www.nerdfitness.com/blog/how-to-become-a-morning-person/

http://www.aasmnet.org/articles.aspx?id=3999

https://hbr.org/2010/07/defend-your-research-the-early-bird-really-does-get-the-worm

http://www.womenshealthmag.com/health/benefits-of-waking-up-early

Alghannam AF, Tsintzas K, Thompson D, Bilzon J, Betts JA. Exploring mechanisms of fatigue during repeated exercise and the dose dependent effects of carbohydrate and protein ingestion: study protocol for a randomized controlled trial. Trials. 2014;15:95. doi: 10.1186/1745-6215-15-95.

Borsheim E, Tipton KD, Wolf SE, Wolfe RR. Essential amino acids and muscle protein recovery from resistance exercise. *Am J Physiol Endocrinol Metab* 2002;283: E648– 57.

Cagney K M. Flexible Dieting 2.0: A flexible nutrition philosophy for the modern athlete. 2016.

Compher C, Frankenfield D, Keim N, Roth-Yousey L, Evidence Analysis Working Group Best practice methods to apply to measurement of resting metabolic rate in adults: a systematic review. J Am Diet Assoc.2006;106:881–903. doi: 10.1016/j.jada.2006.02.009.

Israetel M, Case J, Hoffman J. The Renaissance Diet: A scientific approach to getting leaner and building muscle. Electronic version.

Moore DR, Robinson MJ, Fry JL, Tang JE, Glover EI, Wilkinson SB, Prior T, Tarnopolsky MA, Phillips SM. Ingested protein dose response of muscle and albumin protein synthesis after resistance exercise in young men. Am J Clin Nutr. 2009;89:161–168. doi: 10.3945/ajcn.2008.26401.

Tang JE, Moore DR, Kujbida GW, Tarnopolsky MA, Phillips SM. Ingestion of whey hydrolysate, casein, or soy protein isolate: effects on mixed muscle protein synthesis at rest and following resistance exercise in young men. J Appl Physiol. 2009;107:987–992. doi: 10.1152/japplphysiol.00076.2009.

Tsintzas K, Norton L, Chokkalingam K, Nizamani N, Cooper S, Stephens F, Billeter R, Bennett A. Independent and combined effects of acute physiological hyperglycaemia and hyperinsulinaemia on metabolic gene expression in human skeletal muscle. Clin Sci (Lond) 2013;124:675–684. doi: 10.1042/CS20120481.

Studies on the effectiveness of sprinting

Chan, H., Burns, S. Oxygen consumption, substrate oxidation, and blood pressure following sprint interval exercise. Applied Physiology, Nutrition, and Metabolism. 2013. 38(2), 182-187.

Heydari, M., et al. The effect of high-intensity intermittent exercise on body composition of overweight young males. Journal of Obesity. 2012. 480467. doi: 10.1155/2012/480467.

Smith, A., et al. Dihydrotestosterone is elevated following sprint exercise in healthy young men. Journal of Applied Physiology. 2013. 114(10), 1435-1440.

Esbjornsson, M., et al. Greater growth hormone and insulin response in women than in men during repeated bouts of sprint exercise. Acta Physiology. 2009. 197(2), 107-115.

Winter, B., et al. High impact running improves learning. Neurobiology, Learning, and Memory. 2007. 87(4):597-609.

Schuenke, M., Mikat, R., et al. Effect of an Acute Period of Resistance Exercise on EPOC Implications for Body Mass Management. 2002. 86, 411-417.

Hottenrott, K., Sebastian, L., et al. Effects of High-Intensity Training and Continuous Endurance Training on Aerobic Capacity and Body Composition in Recreationally Active Runners. Journal of Sports Science and Medicine. 2012. 11, 483-488.

Trapp, E., Chisholm, D., et al. The Effects of High-Intensity Intermittent Exercise Training on Fat Loss and Fasting Insulin Levels of Young Women. International Journal of Obesity. 2008. 32(4), 684-691.

Tremblay, A., Simoneau, J., et al. Impact of Exercise Intensity on Body Fatness and Skeletal Muscle Metabolism. Metabolism. 1994. 43(7), 814-818.

Gunnarson, T., Bangsbo, J. The 10-20-30 Training Concept Improves Performance and Health Profile in Moderately Trained Runners. Journal of Applied Physiology. 2012. 113, 1, 1624-1633.

Heydari, M., Freud, J., et al. The Effect of High-Intensity Intermittent Exercise on Body Composition of Overweight Young Males. Journal of Obesity. 2012. Published Ahead of Print.

Tanner, A., Nielsen, B., et al. Salivary Steroid Hormone Response in Trained Men to Running and Circuit Training Sessions. British Journal of Sports Medicine. December 2011. 45(15), A6.

Meckel, Y., Nemet, D., Bar-Sela, S., Radom-Aizik, S. Hormonal and Inflammatory Responses to Different Types of Sprint Interval Training. Journal of Strength and Conditioning Research. 2011. 25(8), 2161-2169.

Irving, B., Davis, C., et al. Effect of Exercise Training Intensity on Abdominal Visceral Fat and Body Composition. Medicine and Science in Sports and Exercise. 2008. 40(11), 1863-1872.

Boudou, P., Sobnngwi, E., et al. Absence of Exercise-Induced Variations in Adiponectin Levels Despite Decreased abdominal Adiposity and Improved Insulin sensitivity in Type 2 Diabetic Men. European Journal of Endocrinology. 2003. 149(5), 421-424.

Macpherson, R., Hazell, T., et al. Run Sprint Interval Training Improves Aerobic Performance but Not Maximal Cardiac Output. Medicine and Science in Sports and Exercise. 2011. 43(1), 115-121.

Strasser, B., Arvandi, M., et al. Resistance training, Visceral Obesity and Inflammatory Response: A Review of the Evidence. Obesity Reviews. 2012. Published Ahead of Print.

Ismail, I., Keating, S., et al. A Systematic Review and Meta-Analysis of the Effect of Aerobic Vs. Resistance Exercise Training on Visceral Fat. Obesity Reviews. 2012. 13, 68-91.

Schuenke, M., Mikat, R., et al. Effect of an Acute Period of Resistance Exercise on EPOC Implications for Body Mass Management. 2002. 86, 411-417.

Appendix 11 studies that show running screws up your thyroid hormones

1. Baylor LS, Hackney AC. Resting thyroid and leptin hormone changes in women following intense, prolonged exercise training. Eur J Appl Physiol. 2003 Jan;88(4-5):480-4.
2. Boyden TW, Pamenter RW, Rotkis TC, Stanforth P, Wilmore JH. Thyroidal changes associated with endurance training in women. Med Sci Sports Exerc. 1984 Jun;16(3):243-6.
3. Wesche MF, Wiersinga WM. Relation between lean body mass and thyroid volume in competition rowers before and during intensive physical training. Horm Metab Res. 2001 Jul;33(7):423-7.
4. Tremblay A, Poehlman ET, Despres JP, Theriault G, Danforth E, Bouchard C. Endurance training with constant energy intake in identical twins: changes over time in energy expenditure and related hormones. Metabolism. 1997 May;46(5):499-503.
5. Rone JK, Dons RF, Reed HL. The effect of endurance training on serum triiodothyronine kinetics in man: physical conditioning

marked by enhanced thyroid hormone metabolism. Clin Endocrinol (Oxf). 1992 Oct;37(4):325-30.

6. Loucks AB, Callister R. Induction and prevention of low-T3 syndrome in exercising women. Am J Physiol. 1993 May;264(5 Pt 2):R924-30.

7. Loucks AB, Heath EM. Induction of low-T3 syndrome in exercising women occurs at a threshold of energy availability. Am J Physiol. 1994 Mar;266(3 Pt 2):R817-23.

8. Rosolowska-Huszcz D. The effect of exercise training intensity on thyroid activity at rest. J Physiol Pharmacol. 1998 Sep;49(3):457-66.

9. Wirth A, Holm G, Lindstedt G, Lundberg PA, Bjorntorp P. Thyroid hormones and lipolysis in physically trained rats. Metabolism. 1981 Mar;30(3):237-41.

10. Opstad PK, Falch D, Oktedalen O, Fonnum F, Wergeland R. The thyroid function in young men during prolonged exercise and the effect of energy and sleep deprivation. Clin Endocrinol (Oxf). 1984 Jun;20(6):657-69.

11. Hohtari H, Pakarinen A, Kauppila A. Serum concentrations of thyrotropin, thyroxine, triiodothyronine and thyroxine binding globulin in female endurance runners and joggers. Acta Endocrinol (Copenh). 1987 Jan;114(1):41-6.

Additional References by URL:

References:

https://www.yahoo.com/health/this-is-what-happens-when-you-stop-exercising-113355357618.html
http://www.cdc.gov/obesity/data/adult.html
http://healthyamericans.org/obesity/
http://www.bodybuilding.com/fun/mohr89.htm
http://www.bodybuilding.com/fun/water.htm
http://www.webmd.com/diet/features/6-reasons-to-drink-water
http://www.mindbodygreen.com/0-4287/10-Reasons-Why-You-Should-Drink-More-Water.html
http://www.bodybuilding.com/fun/clark2.htm
http://articles.mercola.com/sites/articles/archive/2010/11/29/recommended-vegetable-list.aspx
http://www.rd.com/slideshows/healthiest-vegetables/
http://wallstcheatsheet.com/life/gone-green-the-top-10-healthiest-vegetables.html/?a=viewall
http://authoritynutrition.com/11-most-nutrient-dense-foods-on-the-planet/
http://www.whfoods.com/foodstoc.php
http://www.businessinsider.com/41-most-nutritious-fruits-and-vegetables-2014-6
http://www.besthealthmag.ca/eat-well/nutrition/10-of-the-worlds-most-nutritious-foods
http://www.prevention.com/food/healthy-eating-tips/50-healthiest-foods-women
http://www.webmd.com/food-recipes/features/coffee-new-health-food
http://www.eatingwell.com/blogs/health_blog/5_bad_foods_you_should_be_eating
http://fitbie.msn.com/eat-right/tips/5-unhealthy-foods-are-healthier-you-think
http://blogs.laweekly.com/squidink/2011/11/eat_more_pork_8_reasons_why_its_good_for_you.php
http://articles.mercola.com/sites/articles/archive/2011/05/21/why-you-need-to-avoid-low-fat-milk-and-cheese.aspx
http://stronglifts.com/build-muscle-on-a-budget-the-10-cheapest-sources-of-protein/
http://stronglifts.com/20-simple-ways-to-eat-healthy-on-a-budget/

http://www.sharpshopper.net/Documents/Product_Dating.pdf
http://www.helpguide.org/life/healthy_eating_on_budget.htm
http://www.fitsugar.com/Best-Healthy-Food-Shopping-Apps-24768319#/Best-Healthy-Food-Shopping-Apps-24768319?slide=6&image_nid=24768320
http://greatist.com/connect/how-to-move-more-at-work
http://www.sparkpeople.com/blog/blog.asp?post=rise_and_shine_8_stretches_you_should_do_each_morning
http://greatist.com/fitness/kelly-starrett-mobility-injury-free
http://breakingmuscle.com/yoga/increase-strength-by-integrating-yoga-10-essential-postures-for-strength-athletes
http://greatist.com/move/yoga-mega-inflexible-people

National Heart, Blood, and Lung Institute (2005) Replacing Some Carbohydrates with Protein and Unsaturated Fat May Enhance Heart Health Benefits. Retrieved from: http://www.nhlbi.nih.gov/news/press-releases/2005/replacing-some-carbohydrates-with-protein-and-unsaturated-fat-may-enhance-heart-health-benefits

http://www.ncbi.nlm.nih.gov/pubmed/12566476 -- J Nutr. 2003 Feb;133(2):411-7.

Layman DK1, Boileau RA, Erickson DJ, Painter JE, Shiue H, Sather C, Christou DD.

http://www.ncbi.nlm.nih.gov/pubmed/23107521

Resources from Total Health and Fitness Makeover (which served as a guide for this book)
Source on BAC at .05 being major -- (Ferrara, Zancaner, & Georgetti, 1994;Moskowitz & Fiorentino, 2000; Moskowitz, Burns, Fiorentino, Smiley, & Zador, 2000)

Horne, J. A., & Reyner, L. A. (1995). Sleep related vehicle accidents. *BMJ : British Medical Journal*, *310*(6979), 565–567.

Williamson, A., & Feyer, A. (2000). Moderate sleep deprivation produces impairments in cognitive and motor performance equivalent to legally prescribed levels of alcohol intoxication. *Occupational and Environmental Medicine*, *57*(10), 649–655. doi:10.1136/oem.57.10.649

Leger D. The cost of sleep-related accidents: a report for the National Commission on Sleep Disorders Research. Sleep. 1994 Feb;17(1):84–93.

Mitler MM, Carskadon MA, Czeisler CA, Dement WC, Dinges DF, Graeber RC. Catastrophes, sleep, and public policy: consensus report. Sleep. 1988 Feb;11(1):100–109.

Dement WC. The perils of drowsy driving. N Engl J Med. 1997 Sep 11;337(11):783–784.

Howat P, Sleet D, Smith I. Alcohol and driving: is the 0.05% blood alcohol concentration limit justified? Drug Alcohol Rev. 1991;10(2):151–166.

Dawson D, Reid K. Fatigue, alcohol and performance impairment. Nature. 1997 Jul 17;388(6639):235–235.

Johns MW. A new method for measuring daytime sleepiness: the Epworth sleepiness scale. Sleep.1991 Dec;14(6):540–545.

Haraldsson PO, Carenfelt C, Tingvall C. Sleep apnea syndrome symptoms and automobile driving in a general population. J Clin Epidemiol. 1992 Aug;45(8):821–825.

Durnin JV, Womersley J. Body fat assessed from total body density and its estimation from skinfold thickness: measurements on 481 men and women aged from 16 to 72 years. Br J Nutr. 1974 Jul;32(1):77–97.

Pilcher JJ, Huffcutt AI. Effects of sleep deprivation on performance: a meta-analysis. Sleep. 1996 May;19(4):318–326.

Soter NA, Wasserman SI, Austen KF. Cold urticaria: release into the circulation of histamine and eosinophil chemotactic factor of anaphylaxis during cold challenge. N Engl J Med. 1976 Mar 25;294(13):687–690.

Additonal Sleep References:

Dr. Deborah -- http://www.drdeborahmd.com/wise-sleep-solutions

Yoga -- Appl Psychophysiol Biofeedback. 2004 Dec;29(4):269-78.

Treatment of chronic insomnia with yoga: a preliminary study with sleep-wake diaries.

Khalsa SB1.

http://www.urmc.rochester.edu/news/story/index.cfm?id=2866

Made in United States
North Haven, CT
10 November 2026

22091359R00143